Treatment of Diabetes
with Traditional Chinese Medicine

Written By   Chen Jinding
Translated By   Sun Yingkui
                            Zhou Shuhui
English Revised By   Lu Yubin

Shandong Science and Technology Press

Treatment of Diabetes
with Traditional Chinese Medicine

Written by   Chao Jinjing
Translated by   Sun Yuhua
Zhou Shuhai
English Revised by   Lu Yubin

Shandong Science and Technology Press

Preface

Recently, diabetes has become one of the main life-threatening diseases. Since the creation of insulin, great achievements have been obtained in the treatment of the critical and severe cases. As a consequence, the prognosis of the disease is not so severe as before and the patients' lives are prolonged. However, as diabetes is a chronic condition that requires life-long treatment, with a large number of complications, accompanying symptoms and rather complicated clinical manifestations, it is difficult to obtain satisfactory effects with pure Western medicine therapies. Treatment of the disease with TCM, well-known far and wide, is an effective method that can rapidly relieve the symptoms of the disease, and throughout ages, TCM doctors made a lot of expositions on the disease. Considering that there are only a few books that discuss completely and systematically the treatment of the disease with TCM by now, the author, based on the predecessors' and her own years of clinical experience, the experimental studies and the relevant books, summarized the treatment of the disease with TCM and wrote the book, for the reference of the doctors engaging in the research, prevention and treatment of the disease and the patients conducting treatment, prevention, nursing and observation themselves.

Under the guidance of the theory of both the Western medicine and the traditional Chinese medicine, this book chiefly expounds the method to treat diabetes and its main complications, currently commonly-used therapies for different types of the disease and the law to select drugs and formulas according to zang-fu theory, and introduces the commonly-used and effective Chinese herbs and formulas that can reduce sugar content in blood. In special chapters, the treatment of the main complications and the senile diabetes are intro-

1

duced.

This book, with its rich contents and systemic introduction to the knowledge on the treatment of the disease with TCM, is a useful book to both doctors and patients.

Chen Jinding

2

CONTENTS

Chapter 1 Introduction 1

　1. 1 Definition 2

　1. 2 Discussion of the ancients on Xiaoke Syndrome 3

　1. 3 A survey of the study of diabetes in modern times 5

Chapter 2 Causes and Pathogenesis 16

　2. 1 Causes and pathogenesis 16

　2. 2 The law of occurrence of diabetes 19

　2. 3 The characteristics of pathogenesis 22

Chapter 3 Syndrome Identification

　　　　and Corresponding Treatment 26

　3. 1 Essentials of syndrome identification 27

　3. 2 Essentials of treatment 29

　3. 3 Syndromes identification

　　　　and corresponding treatment 31

　3. 4 The commonly-used therapeutic methods 90

Chapter 4 Classifications of the Commonly-used

　　　　Formulas and Herbs 95

　4. 1 The commonly-used Chinese herbs in clinic 95

　4. 2 The commonly-used formulas in clinic 102

　4. 3 The commonly-used simple and proved formulas 114

Chapter 5 Diabetes in the Aged 119

　5. 1 Prevention and treatment of senile diabetes 120

　5. 2 TCM treatment of senile diabetes 121

　5. 3 Case study 132

Chapter 6 Diagnosis and Treatment of

　　　　Gravidic Diabetes 136

　6. 1 Syndrome identification and corresponding

treatment of gravidic diabetes ································ 137

6. 2 Recuperation after delivery ····························· 140

6. 3 Case study ·· 142

Chapter 7 Common Clinical Complications of Diabetes ········· 144

7. 1 Diabetes nephrosis ····································· 144

7. 2 Diabetes and hypertension ······························ 155

7. 3 Diabetic retinal lesion ·································· 165

7. 4 Diabetes complicated with ketosis ······················ 171

7. 5 Diabetes complicated by acrometic

necrosis(diabetic foot) ·································· 179

7. 6 Diabetes complicated by impotence ····················· 188

Chapter 8 Diet Therapy and Medicated Diet ···················· 197

8. 1 Single drug or food ···································· 197

8. 2 Commonly used formulas ······························· 199

Chapter 9 Other Therapies of Traditional Chinese Medicine ··· 203

9. 1 Qigong therapy ··· 203

9. 2 Acupuncture therapy ···································· 210

9. 3 Massage therapy ·· 218

Chapter 1　Introduction

Diabetes is a systemic and chronic disease concerning the metabolic disturbance and the disorders of the endocrine system. It is divided into two types: the primary and the secondary. Most of the disease are the former type. Its etiologic factors and pathologic mechanism is still not clear enough, maybe concerning with hereditary factors, virus infection, autoimmunity or hyperglucogen. But its basic physiopathologic mechanism is the absolute or relative hypoinsulinism, which results in the metabolic disturbance of the sugar, protein, fat, water and electrolyte, or even the acid-base imbalance. This disease is characterized by hyperglycemia, increased urine sugar, sugar tolerance reduction and abnormal insulin release. Clinically, it is usually asymptomatic at the early stage. When it develops further, it may present polyphagia, polydipsia, polyuria, severe thirst, easy to be hunger, emaciation, and lassitude, or even gives rise to the complications of the cardiovascular system, the kidney, the eyes and the nerves in a chronic case. In severe cases or in a stress state, the patients may undergo ketoacidosis, hypertonic coma and lactic acidosis, which often lead to death, and may develop such complications as pyogenic infection, urinary infection, mycotid infection or pulmonary tuberculosis. Most of the patients would die of the complication of the cardiovascular system. However, if the disease is positively prevented and treated earlier, the patients may be generally good and their strength may be restored to normal.

Diabetes in Western medicine is basically consistent with Xiaoke Syndrome in TCM according to their manifestations. Therefore, diabetes may be included in Xiaoke Syndrome, which is a morbid state caused by improper diet and emotional disturbance and marked by

1

polydipsia, polyphagia, polyuria, emaciation or the urine tasting sweet. Knowledge to diabetes in China occurs most earliest in the world. In the great medical book the *Yellow Emperor's Internal Classic* written in 400 B. C. , there were already detailed descriptions on the disease. In recent years, with the advancement of TCM, treatment of diabetes with TCM has been loved by the vast patients and has achieved ideally effects.

1. 1 Definition

Xiaoke Syndrome (diabetes) is a disease characterized by polydipsia, polyphagia, polyuria and the urine of sweet taste.

There is not yet a clear definition about diabetes in Western medicine. Most doctors believe that it is a disease of endocrine metabolism abnormality and a syndrome with impairment of multiple systems and visceral organs mainly marked by persistent hyperglycemia due to absolute or relative inadequate secretion of insulin. It is a common and life-long disease which may cause specific disturbance of the microcirculation and arteriosclerosis of the great vessels. According to the statistics in a survey report on the diabetics among 30, 000 populations in 14 provinces of China, the incidence of the disease is 6. 74% and has an increasing tendency. During the application of oral antihyperglycemia, it has been found that the Western drugs may promote the occurrence of the cardiocerebral complications. So, many doctors adevocate that TCM should be adopted to treat the disease. Although Western medicine and TCM name the disease differently, their descriptions and therapeutic purpose on the disease are about the same. For this reason, diabetes in Western medicine can be diagnosed and treated in TCM based on the laws of Xiaoke Syndrome. Even better therapeutic effect can be expected if both Chinese and Western therapies are applied in accordance with the result of the syndrome identification of TCM and that of Western diagnosis and early treatment is given. For mild and moderate dia-

2

betes, TCM therapy not only can relieve the symptoms, but also can prevent and delay the occurrence of the complications and the concommitant diseases. Therefore, it is a new way for the treatment of diabetes.

1.2 Discussion of the ancients on Xiaoke Syndrome

This disease is named Xiaodan in the *Yellow Emperor's Internal Classic*, or Xiao, Gexiao, Feixiao and Xiaozhong in accordance with its different pathogenesis and different manifestations. It was also pointed out in *On Miraculous Disease*, a chapter of the *Plain Questions of the Yellow Emperor's Internal Classic*, that "diabetics must have eaten so much sweet and fat food that they are usually very fat. Fat food leads to accumulated heat in the interior, while the sweet food often produces accumulation in the middle-jiao. If the accumulated heat and the stagnancy go upwards, Xiaoke Syndrome will occur as a result." It is clear that at that time the relation between intake of the high caloric food and the occurrence of diabetes has been realized. The doctors through the ages advanced the study of this disease on the basis of the *Yellow Emperor's Internal Classic*. In the book *Synopsis of Prescriptions of the Golden Chamber*, for example, there was a treatise entitled on *The Manifestations and Treatment of Xiaoke Syndrome, Dysuria and Stranguria*, in which Xiaoke, as a name of disease, was put forward and discussed. It was stated that "A diabetic patient may urinate as much as he drinks, this condition should be treated with Shenqi Wan (Bolus for Tonifying the Kidney-qi)", which involves polyuria; that "Those with severe thirst and intake of much water are treated with Wenge San (Powder of Gecko)", which refers to polydipsia, and that "Those with desire for drink and dry mouth and tongue should be treated with Baihu Jia Renshen Tang (White Tiger Decoction with Ginseng)", which indicates the symptoms of severe thirst and dry mouth and tongue in diabetics. In this treatise the symptoms and the formulas and herbs for the treatment of the three

3

types of Xiaoke Syndrome were also mentioned. In the chapter of Xiaoke Syndrome of the book *Treatise on the Causes and Symptoms of Diseases*, Xiaoke Syndrome was used as a general term for various types of the disease and was exactly defined, remarking that "Xiaoke Syndrome is a disease marked by persistent thirst with polyuria". As for its development, it was stated that "carbuncles and other complications may occur". Wang Tao in the Tang Dynasty, quoted from the *Ancient and Modern Medical Experience* that: "thirst with desire for drinking, freuqent urination with suspension and a sweet taste of bran indicate Xiaoke Syndrome" in the chapter of Xiaozhong (diabetes with polyphgia as the prominent symptom), Xiaoke (diabetes with polydipsia as the prominent symptom) and Shenxiao (diabetes mainly involving the kidney) in the book *Secrets of an Official*. He also pointed out that "everytime this disease comes on, the urine must be sweet", and that "diabetics will become emaciated". In the book *The Precious Mirror of Hygiene*, it said that "those who have Xiaoke Syndrome frequently urinate with the color of the urine as dark as that of oil, the suspension of the urine as sweet as honey". This showed that the ancient Chinese had had further understanding of the clinical characteristic of Xiaoke Syndrome by that time. The ancient Chinese knew that the urine was sweet by their tongues. This might be a quanlitative change of the understanding of the disease, which occurs red earlier than that in other countries, 1 000 years earlier than Englishman Willis Thomas(1672), who found and named the disease after the urine as sweet as honey. There were also many expositions on the complications of the disease. For example, in the book *Confucious Duties to Their Parents*, the author said: "many of the patients suffering from diabetes become deaf and blind, and have sore, tinea, furuncle, etc. " or "have hectic fever and sweet due to debility and cough due to deficiency of the lung". The doctors in the later generations classified Xiaoke Syndrome as three types, Shangxiao (diabetes involving the upper- jiao), Zhongxiao (diabetes involving the middle-jiao) and Xiaxiao (diabetes involving the lower-jiao) according to the seriousness of the three major symptoms of polydipsia, polyphagia and polyuria. In the chapter of Xiaodan of the book *Standards of Diagnosis and Treatment*, for example, the author wrote: "Feeling thirst and frequent drinking indicates Shangxiao; polyphagia indicates Zhongxiao; and polyuria with thick suspension associated with severe thirst indicates Xiaxiao". It has been believed that the three types could not be absolutely isolated in the treatment. As was pointed out in the chapter of Xiaoke Syndrome Category of the book *General Collection for Holy Relief*. "According to the cause, the three types are the same, while according to their manifestations, they are different". Generally speaking, understanding of the disease in TCM has a long history, is of a distant source and a long stream. The theory on the disease is derived from the *Yellow Emperor's Internal Classic*, its diagnosis and treatment from the *Synopsis of Prescriptions of the Golden Chamber*, its classification from the *General Treatise on the Causes and Symptoms of Diseases*. To sum up, the contents on the theory of Xiaoke Syndrome in the ancient medical literature are quite abundant, which provides us with valuable data for studying the disease today.

1. 3 A survey of the study of diabetes in modern times

In modern times a large number of clinical and experimental studies on diabetes have been made based on the theory of Xiaoke Syndrome in TCM. The contents can be classified as the following parts:

1. 3. 1 Clinical study of the types and syndromes classification

As diabetes is a group of chronic metabolic disease with multiple manifestations and complicated conditions, its cause remains unknown by now and there is no unified standard for evaluation of treatment. Having fought against the disease for a long time, the modern doctors have accumulated a wealth of experience. They have also achieved rich experience and achievements through performing diagnosis and treatment on the basis of both the features of TCM in treating the disease and the Concept of Wholism in TCM.

1) The severn types classified by Zhu Chenyu

Having combined doctor Shi Jinmo's clinical experience, Zhu observed more than 1,000 cases and systemactically summarized the index for different types and syndromes of the disease and the corresponding treatment schedules by adopting the method of combining the syndrome diagnosis and the disease diagnosis.

(1) Type of yin-deficiency

Therapeutic method: nourishing yin and promoting the production of the body fluid, assisted by activating the blood flow.

Prescription: Bei Sha Shen (Radix Glehniae) 10g, Mai Dong (Radix Ophiopogonis) 10g, Gou Qi Zi (Fructus Lycii) 10g, Dang Gui (Radix Angelicae Sinensis) 10g, Chuan Lian Zi (Fructus Meliae Toosensan) 10g, Sheng Di (Radix Rehmanniae) 15g, Shu Di (Radix Rehmanniae Praeparata) 15g, Ge Gen (Radix Puerariae) 15g, Dan Shen (Radix Salviae Miltiorrhizae) 30g.

(2) Type of hyperactivity of fire due to yin-deficiency

Therapeutic method: nourishing yin to reduce fire, assisted by activating blood flow.

Prescription: The above recipe with the drugs clearing away heat added (the heat-clearing drugs should be added according to the results of syndrome identification in accordance with the theory of zang-fu organs).

(3) Type of deficiency of both qi and yin

Therapeutic method: supplementing qi and nourishing yin, supported by activating the blood flow.

Prescription: Huang Qi (Radix Astragali seu Hedysari) 30g, Xuan Shen (Radix Scrophulariae) 30g, Dan Shen (Radix Salviae Miltiorrhizae) 30g, Mu Li (Concha Ostreae) 30g, Shan Yao (Rhizoma Dioscoree) 10g, Dang Shen (Radix Codonopsis Pilosula) 10g, Mai Dong (Radix Ophiopogonis) 10g, Wu Wei Zi (Fructus Schisandrae) 10g, Cang Zhu (Rhizoma Atractylodis) 15g, Sheng Di (Radix

6

Rehmanniae) 15g, Shu Di (Radix Rehmanniae Praeparata) 15g, Ge Gen (Radix Puerariae)15g,Fu Ling (Poria)15g.

(4) Type of deficiency of both qi and yin and exuberance of fire

Therapeutic method: supplementing qi, nourishing yin and reducing fire,assisted by activating blood flow.

Prescription: the same as that for type (3), to which heat-clearing drugs should be added according to the patients' condition deliberately.

(5)Type of Deficiency of both yin and yang

Therapeutic method: warming up yang and nourishing yin, supported by activating blood flow.

Prescription: Gui Zhi (Ramulus Cinnamomi)10g,Shan Yao (Rhizoma Dioscoreae)10g, Shan Yu Rou (Fructus Corni) 10g, Dan Pi (Cortex Moutan Radicis) 10g, Ze Xie (Rhizoma Alismatis) 10g, Sheng Di (Radix Rehmanniae) 15g, Shu Di (Radix Rehmanniae Praeparata) 15g, Fu Ling (Poria) 15g, Ge Gen (Radix Puerariae) 15g, Zhi Fu Zi(Radix Aconiti Praeparata)5g.

(6) Type of deficieny of yin and yang and exuberance of fire

Therapeutic method: warming up yang, nourishing yin and reducing fire, assisted by activating blood flow.

Prescription: the recipe for type (5) to which Zhi Mu (Rhizoma Anemarrhenae)10g and Huang Bai (Cortex Phellodendri) 10g are added.

(7) Type of blood stasis

Therapeutic method: activating flow of both blood and qi, assisted by treating the primary cause of the disease.

Prescription: Mu Xiang (Radix Aucklandiae) 10g, Dang Gui (Radix Angelicae Sinensis) 10g, Chuan Xiong (Rhizoma Ligustici Chuanxiong) 10g, Yi Mu Cao (Herba Leonuri) 30g, Dan Shen (Radix Salviae Miltiorrhizae) 30g, Chi Shao (Radix Paeoniae Rubra) 15g, Ge Gen (Radix Puerariae) 15g, Sheng Di (Radix Rehmanniae)15g, Shu Di (Radix Rehamnniae Praeparata)15g.

2) The five stages classified by Lu Renhe

Stage I (Stage of yin-deficiency):

Clinical manifestations: strong physique, full of vim and vigour, lowered endurance, red tongue with yellow coating, mild hyperglycemia and hyperlipoidemia, absence of the urine sugar.

This stage can exhibit two kinds of different syndromes: the syndrome of yin-deficiency and hyperactivity of the liver, which should be treated by nourishing yin and softening the liver; and that of hyperactivity of yang due to yin- deficiency, which should be treated by nourishing yin to suppress the hyperactive yang.

Stage II (stage of heat transmission):

Clinical manifestations: aversion to heat and desire for cold, polyuria, polydipsia, polyphagia, lassitude and emaciation, elevation of both the blood sugar and the urine sugar.

This stage may present four kinds of different syndromes: the syndrome of accumulation of heat in the Yangming meridian, which should be treated by clearing away heat from the Yangming meridian; that of toxic heat in the lung, which should be treated by clearing away heat from the lung and removing toxic materials; that of stagnation of the liver qi producing heat, which should be treated by relieving the depression of the liver and clearing away heat; and that of spleen deficiency complicated with dampness-heat, which should be treated by strengthening the spleen to remove dampness and clearing away heat by inducing diuresis.

Stage III (the stage of dryness-heat impairing yin and inactiveness of qi in the meridians):

Clinical manifestations: dry mouth and tongue, soreness and weakness of the loins and knees, pain of the limbs, lassitude, dark red tongue, elevation of the blood sugar and the urine sugar, and tendency to present complications.

This stage may be manifested as six kinds of different syndromes: the syndrome of dryness-heat imparing the kidney and injury of both

8

qi and yin, which should be treated by tonifying the kidney, supplementing qi, nourishing yin and moistening dryness; that of malnutrition of the meridians due to dryness- heat impairing yin, which should be treated mainly by promoting circulation of qi and blood in the meridians and collaterals; that of impairment of yin by dryness-heat involving both the lung and the spleen, which should be treated by tonifying qi, strengthening the spleen, clearing away heat and moistening the lung; that of dryness-heat and impairment of yin involving the heart and the spleen, which should be treated by tonifying the kidney and supplementing qi aided by treating the heart and the spleen; that of dryness-heat and impairment of yin accompanied with stagnancy in the middle-jiao, which should be treated by regulating the function of the middle- jiao, supplementing qi, clearing away heat and removing the stagnancy; and that of dryness-heat and impairment of yin accompanied with liver depression and blood stasis, which should be treated by supplementing qi, promoting the circulation of blood and relieving the liver depression.

Stage IV (The stage of deficiency of yin, yang and qi, and obstruction of the meridians):

Clinical manifestations: aversion to both cold and heat, listlessness, lassitude, soreness, pain and debility of the limbs, tendons and bones, unstable blood sugar, and aggravation of the complications.

This stage may present four kinds of different syndromes: the syndrome of obstruction of the meridians, which should be treated by harmonizing yin and yang, promoting blood flow and removing obstruction of the meridans; that of loss of nourishment of meridians, which should be treated by stregthening the spleen and nourishing the liver; that of malnutrition of the urogenital region, which should be treated by supplementing qi, benifiting the kidney, supporting yang and strengthening tendons; and that of loss of nourishment of the stomach and intestine, which should be treated by moistening the intestine to loose bowel in the case of dry stool and strengthening the spleen to stop diarrhea in the case of loose stool.

Stage V (Stage of critical and severe stage of the complications):

The complications must be treated emergently under the coordination of the doctors from the related medical fields, otherwise, the patients may be disabled or die.

3) The seven types classified by Jiang Tianyou

(1) The type of deficiency of both qi and yin

This type can be treated with combined Huangqi Tang (Astragalus Root Decoction)and Zengye Tang (Fluid- increasing Decoction) with modifications, and the ingredients are:

Huang Qi (Radix Astragali seu Hedysari) 15g, Dang Shen(Radix Codonopsis Pilosula) 9g, Shan Yao(Rhizoma Dioscoreae)15g, Gan Cao(Radix Glycyrrhizae) 6g, Xuan Shen(Radix Scrophulariae) 9g, Mai Dong(Radix Ophiopogonis) 15g, Tian Dong(Radix Asparagi) 9g, Zhi Mu (Rhizoma Anemarrhenae) 15g, Hua Fen (Radix Trichosanthis) 9g, Shu Di(Radix Rehmanniae Praeparata)9g, and Gou Qi(Fructus Lycii) 12g.

(2) The type of stagnation of dampness-heat

This type can be treated with Ganlu Xiaodu Dan (Sweet Dew Detoxication Pill) with modifications, the ingredients of which are:

Bai Kou Ren (Semen Amomi Gardamomi) 9g,Huo Xiang (Herba Agastachis)9g, Yin Chen (Herba Artemisiae Capillaris)9g,Hua Shi (Talcum)15g, Mu Tong(Caulis Akebiae) 6g, Shi Chang Pu(Rhizoma Acori Graminei) 4.5g, Huang Qin(Radix Scutellariae) 9g, Zhe Bei (Bulbus Fritillariae Thunbergii) 9g, Lian Qiao (Fructus Forsythiae) 9g, She Gan(Rhizoma Belamcandae) 9g, Bo He(Herba Menthae) 6g, Da Huang(Radix seu Rhizoma Rhei) 9g, and Zhi Mu (Rhizoma Anemarrhenae) 9g.

(3) The type of unconsolidation due to yang-deficiency

This type can be treated with Jinkui Shenqi Wan (Bolus of Golden Chamber for Tonifying the Kidney-qi)with modifications, the ingredients of which are:

10

Shu Di(Radix Rehmanniae Praeparata) 12g, Shan Yu Rou(Fructus Corni) 9g, Shan Yao(Rhizoma Dioscoreae) 30g, Dan Pi(Cortex Moutan Radicis) 9g, Fu Ling (Poria) 9g, Ze Xie (Rhizoma Alismatis) 6g, Rou Gui(Cortex Cinnamomi) 9g, Fu Zi (Radix Aconiti Praeparata) 9g, Fu Pen Zi(Fructus Rubi) 12g, and Tian Hua Fen(Radix Trichosanthis) 15g.

(4)The type of inability to astringe due to yin-deficiency

This type can be treated with combined Liuwei Dihuang Tang(Decoction of Six Drugs with Rehmannia Root) and Wuzi Yanzong Wan (Pill of Seeds of Five Drugs for Treating Masculin Sterility) with modifications. Its ingredients are:

Shu Di(Radix Rehmanniae Praeparata) 12g, Shan Yao(Rhizoma Dioscoreae) 30g, Ze Xie(Rhizoma Alismatis) 6g, Nu Zhen Zi(Fructus Ligustri Lucidi) 15g, Han Lian Cao(Herba Ecliptae) 15g, Gou Qi Zi(Fructus Lycii) 15g, Fu Pen Zi(Fructus Rubi) 15g, Wu Bei Zi (Galla Chinensis) 9g, Jin Ying Zi (Fructus Rosae Laevigatae) 12g, Lian Xu (Stamen Nelumbinis) 15g, Di Gu Pi (Cortex Lycii Radicis) 15g, and Hua Fen(Radix Trichosanthis) 12g.

(5)The type of stagnation of the liver-qi and deficiency of yin

This should be treat first with modified Danzhi Xiaoyao San(Ease Powder of Montan Bark and Cape Jasmine), the ingredients of which are:

Dang Gui(Radix Angelicae Sinensis) 10g, Bai Shao(Radix Paeoniae Alba) 10g, Chai Hu(Radix Bupleuri) 9g, Fu Ling(Poria) 9g, Shan Yao(Rhizoma Dioscoreae) 12g, Xiang Fu(Rhizoma Cyperi) 9g, Dan Pi(Cortex Moutan Radicis) 9g, Zhi Zi(Fructus Gardeniae) 9g, Gou Qi(Fructus Lycii) 10g, He Huan Hua(Flos Albiziae) 15g, Yin Chen(Herba Artemisiae Capillaris) 9g, Di Gu Pi(Cortex Lycii) 30g, Ze Xie(Rhizoma Alismatis) 6g, and Ju Hua(Flos Chrysanthemi) 10g.

When six doses of the above formula are continuously administered, replace it with the formula regulating both the liver and the kidney which consists of the following drugs:

Sheng Di(Radix Rehmanniae) 10g, Xuan Shen(Radix Scrophulariae) 30g, Shan Yao(Rhizoma Dioscoreae) 12g, Dan Pi (Cortex Moutan Radicis)10g, Di Gu Pi(Cortex Lycii) 30g, Hua Fen(Radix Trichosanthis) 30g, Cao Jue Ming(Semen Cassiae) 30g, Dang Gui (Radix Angelicae Sinensis) 9g, Bai Shao (Radix Paeoniae Alba) 12g, Ju Hua (Flos Chrysanthemi)15g, Yu Jin (Radix Curcumae) 9g, Xiang Fu (Rhizoma Cyperi, processed with vinegar) 10g, and Ye Jiao Teng(Caulis Polygoni Multiflori) 30g.

(6) The type of dryness-heat with yin deficiency

This type can be treated with combined Liuwei Dihuang Tang(Decoction of Six Drugs Including Rehmannia Root) and Baihu Tang (White Tiger Decoction) with modifications, which consists of:

Shu Di(Radix Rehmanniae Praeparata) 15g, Shan Yao(Rhizoma Dioscoreae) 15g, Nu Zhen Zi(Fructus Ligustri Lucidi) 15g, Dan Pi (Cortex Moutan Radicis) 10g, Ze Xie(Rhizoma Alismatis) 6g, Fu Ling(Poria)6g, Sheng Shi Gao(Gypsum Fibrosum) 6g, Zhi Mu(Rhizoma Anemarrhenae) 12g, Ban Xia Mo(Powder of Rhizoma Pinelliae) 9g, Tian Hua Fen(Radix Trichosanthis) 30g, Da Huang(Radix seu Rhizoma Rhei,to be decocted later) 12g.

(7) The type of yin-deficiency involving the three portions of triple -jiao.

This type should be treated with combined Ganlu Yin(Sweet Dew Decoction) and Baihu Tang (White Tiger Decoction)with modifications, which are composed of:

Sheng Di(Radix Rehmanniae) 12—15g, Shu Di(Radix Rehmanniae Praeparata) 12—15g, Tian Dong(Radix Adenophorae Strictae) 12—15g, Mai Dong (Radix Ophiopogonis) 12—15g, Huang Qin (Radix Scutellariae) 9g, Tian Hua Fen(Radix Trichosanthis) 30g, Bei Sha Shen(Radix Asparagi) 15—30g, Sheng Shi Gao(Gypsum Fibrosum) 30—150g, Huang Qi(Radix Astragali seu Hedysari) 30g.

To the above drugs, Xuan Shen(Radix Scrophulariae) and Shan

12

Dou Gen (Radix Sophorae Subprostrate)may be added to clear away heat and relieve sore throat, Long Chi(Dens Draconis) to tranquilze the mind, Chen Pi (Pericarpium Citri Reticulatae) to promote the flow of qi, or Dan Shen(Radix Salviae Miltiorrhizae) to activate the blood flow. In the later stage, Wu Wei Zi(Fructus Schisandrae), Sang Ji Sheng(Ramulus Loranthi) and Nu Zhen Zi(Fructus Ligustri Lucidi) should be added to tonify both the liver and the kidney.

1. 3. 2 Using special formulas on the basis of syndrome identification

① Believing that the pathogenesis of diabetes lies in primarily yin deficiency and secondarily the production of dryness- heat, Tian, etc. , treat diabetes mainly with the formulas nourishing yin and clearing away heat which are modified deliberately according to patients' conditions. The commonly-used drugs are as follows:

Tian Hua Fen(Radix Trichosanthis), Sheng Di (Radix Rehmanniae), Shu Di (Radix Rehmanniae Praeparata), Tian Dong (Radix Adenophorae Strictae), Mai Dong(Radix Ophiopogonis), Sheng Shi Gao(Gypsum Fibrosum) , Zhi Mu(Rhizoma Anemarrhenae), Xuan Shen (Radix Scrophulariae), Huang Qi (Radix Astragali seu Hedysari), Wu Wei Zi(Fructus Schsandrae), etc.

Tian treated 215 cases of diabetes with the above method. The results are that 60 cases were almostly cured and the totally effective rate reached 70 percent.

② Teng, etc. , hold that deficiency of both qi and yin are the fundamental pathogenesis of diabetes. So they treat the disease with the formulas with the action of supplementing qi and nourishing yin with modifications according to the patients' conditions. The commonly-used drugs are:

Huang Qi(Radix Astragali seu Hedysari), Ren Shen(Radix Ginseng) or Dang Shen (Radix Codonopsis Pilosulae), Shan Yao(Rhizoma Dioscoreae), Sheng Di(Radix Rehmanniae), Shu Di (Radix Rehmanniae Praeparata), Huang Jing(Rhizoma Polygonati), Gou

13

Qi Zi (Fructus Lycii), Mai Dong (Radix Ophiopogonis), Dan Shen (Radix Salviae Miltiorrhizae), Sheng Shi Gao (Gypsum Fibrosum), etc.

Teng has treated 50 cases of diabetes with a totally effective rate of 82 percent.

③ Leiyunshang Pharmaceutical Factory of Suzhou developed Xiaoke Chongji (Drug Powder for Diabetes to be taken after infused in water) according to Doctor Wang's clinical experience.

④ Wuwei Dihuang Tang (Decoction of Five Drugs with Rehmannia Root) was applied to treat the disease in Beijing College of Traditional Chinese Medicine with satisfactory therapeutic effects.

⑤ Fufang Xiaokeping Pian (Compound Tablets for Treating Diabetes), developed cooperatively in Shandong College of Traditional Chinese Medicine and Yantai Traditional Chinese Herbal Factory, were adopted to treat 333 cases of diabetes with a totally effective rate of 81.1 percent.

⑥ Zhang Fulin applied the TCM drugs with the action of nourishing yin to clear away heat and activating blood flow to remove the obstruction of the collaterals to the treatment of 13 cases of non-insulin-dependent diabetes complicated with diseases of the peripheral verves which didn't respond to the long administered Western drugs. After 4.5—5 months treatment, the patients' symptoms and signs were relieved and the transmission speed of their periphearal nerves was improved.

1.3.3 Study on the effect of simple recipe and compound formulas on the reduction of blood sugar

① Fu reported that Renshen Baihu Tang (White Tiger Decoction with Ginseng can reduce experimental hyperglycemia and relieve the experimental diabetes in rats.

② Wang Zhengang, etc. reported that Ren Shen (Radix Ginseng) can reduce the blood sugar in both normal dogs and alloxan diabetes dogs.

14

③Luo Yuanwei claimed that Ge Gen (Radix Puerariae) can reduce the blood sugar.

④ The study of Fang Qicheng, etc. showed that isoflavone Radix Puerariae Element is the main active ingredient of Ge Gen (Radix Puerariae).

⑤ The influence of the Chinese drug Xiaoke Ping Tablets on the blood sugar of the models of alloxan diabetes mice and normal rabbits was observed in Shandong College of Traditional Chinese Medicine. The experiment showed that the drug can reduce the blood sugar in both experimental mice and normal rabbits.

Chapter 2　Causes and Pathogenesis

　　The causes of the primary diabetes are still not expounded completely, as diabetes is a group of syndromes marked by hyperglycemia rather than a single disease. In recent years, doctors have found through their studies that the occurrence of diabetes is concerned with many factors, the most commonly-encountered heredity, virus infection, obesity and multiparity. In the old people, deficiency of the kidney -qi and the ensuing decline of the pancreas function, if accompanied with obesity, inadequate exercise or excessive intake of sweet food, often lead to elevation of the blood sugar and eventually the occurrence of diabetes. According to TCM, congenital deficiency, improper diet, emotional disturbance, over strain, excessive sexual activities, or overuse of drugs warm in taste and dry in nature all serve as the main causes of the disease.

2. 1 Causes and pathogenesis

1) Improper diet

　　Long-standing excessive intake of fat and sweet, hot, dry and stimulus food or indulgence in alcohol impair the spleen and stomach and, as a result, causes stagnancy in the stomach, which produces heat in the interior. Accumulation of the interior heat may transform into dryness and impair yin, leading to accumulation and stagnation of the dryness and heat in the stomach. As a consequence, the polyphagia is aggravated, and if the organs and meridians losses of moisturization due to impairment of the body fluid, diabetes will occur. In the chapter of Xiaoke Syndrome of the book *Secrets of An Official*, there is a quotation: "Excessive intake of food and alcohol salty or sour in flavor for years may lead to exuberant heat in the triple-jiao and dryness of the five zang organs. In this way, wood and rock will be dried up, let alone the human being?" The chapter of Xiaoke Syndrome of the book *Danxi's Experiential Therapy* also says: "Overdrinking, preference for fried food can, therefore, result in flaring up of fire to produce heat in the viscera. Exuberance of dryness-heat dries the body fluid, so polydipsia occurs. " All this shows that improper diet has a close relationship to the occurrence of the disease. In addition, accumulation of phlegm often happens to the fat men. The stagnated phlegm may produce heat and cause blood stasis, which will in turn consume the body fluid and lead to the subsequent production of dryness-heat. When the dryness-heat forms, it will impair the yin-fluid further, forming a vicious circle which, in the case of existing a long time, will induce the development or aggravation of diabetes. Su Dongpo in the Song Dynasty wrote that overeating fruit would also cause diabetes and he called this kind of diabetes "Fruit Diabetes".

2) Emotional disturbance

Long term emotional disturbance is also responsible for the occurrence of the disease. For example, mental depression impairs the liver and causes stagnation of the liver-qi, which will transform into exuberant fire to go up to consume the yin-fluid of both the lung and the stomach or downward to consume the kidney-yin; in other word, emotional disturbance will cause failure of the liver to perform its dispersing and discharging effect and inability of the kidney to store, as a result, fire flares up and the body fluid in the lower is consumed, resulting in polydipsia, polyphagia and polyuria. In addition, flaring-up of the fire transformed from the stagnated heart-qi will lead to impairment of the essence and blood of the heart and spleen, and the depletion of the kidney-yin in the lower part of the body. This will further cause breakdown of the coordination between the heart and the kidney, giving rise to diabetes. In the book *Confucious Duties to Their Parents*, the author wrote: "In diabetics, exhaustion of the mind and emotional disturbance result in accumulation of exuberant dryness-heat. " The chapter of Three Types of Xiaoke Synrome of the book *A Guide to Clinical Practice with Medical Records* says: "Mental depression will cause fire in the interior from which Xiaoke Syndrome results. " All these indicate that emotional stress that causes stagnation of fire and impairment of yin is an important cause of diabetes.

3) Excessive sexual activities

In the case of congenital yin-deficiency, excessive sexual activities will give rise to consumption of the kidney-essence and the production of fire of the deficiency-type in the interior, which will eventually cause the kidney-deficiency, lung-dryness and stomach-heat, and the ensuing occurrence of diabetes as, a result, the "insufficiency of water leads to excess of fire, and excessive of fire again leads to more insufficiency of the water. " In the chapter of Xiaoke Syndrome of the book *Prescriptions for Emergencies Worthy One Thousand Golds*, it was stated that the Xiaoke Syndrome is caused by "intemperance in sexual life: When the patients were able-bodied, they didn't cherish their health but indulged in sexual pleasures, whereas when they are a bit old, their kidney-qi will be exhausted and deficient. All this is due to intemperance in sexual life. " It was also stated in the chapter of Xiaoke Syndrome of the book *Secrets of An Official* that "Diabetes is caused by excessive sexual activities which result in deficiency of the kidney-qi. Heat produced in the lower-jiao is responsible for the kidney-dryness and the resultant Xiaoke Syndrome. " This shows that intemperance in sexual life and the subsequent kidney-dryness and kidney-essence deficiency have certain relationships to the occurrence of the disease.

4) Congenital deficiency

Weakness of the five zang-organs due to congenital deficiency, especially weakness of the kidney, is related to the occurrence of diabetes. The five zang-organs store the essence which serves as the basis of the life, and the kidney receives the essence from the other or-

18

gans to store. Therefore, when the five zang organs are hypofunctional, they have not enough essence, qi and blood for the kidney to store. In this case, if no proper care is provided, the kidney-essence as well as the body fluid will be exhausted, leading to the development of diabetes. Just as stated in the chapter of Five Changes of the book *Miraculous Pivot*, "those with weakness of the five zang organs are likely to suffer from diabetes."

5) Overuse of drugs of warm and dry nature

Predecessors believed that addition to drugs or pills for strengthening yang would produce dryness-heat to impair yin. Now the atmosphere of taking this kind of drugs has ceased to exist, but it is still not seldom for those who take the warm and dry drugs for the purpose of strengthening yang to live longer or have pleasure, or those who take the drugs erroneously for a long time in the course of their chronic disease, to suffer from diabetes as a result of the production of dryness-heat and depletion of the yin-fluid.

2.2 The law of occurrence of diabetes

1) Pathological changes in zang-fu organs

Diabetes involves all the three portions of the triple-jiao. In the upper, it involves the lung, in the middle, it involves the stomach, and in the lower it involves the kidney. Of the pathologic changes of the organs involved, that of the kidney is the most important.

(1) Pathologic change in the upper-jiao

This refers to dryness impairing the body fluid in the lung. The lung is the upper source of water and regulates the water metabolism. When dryness-heat impairs the lung and disturbs the normal function of the lung, water will be sent down too much to cause polyuria and the lung will fail to distribute the water to cause polydipsia.

Diabetes is mainly marked by deficiency of the lung-qi and lung-dryness in the upper-jiao which lead to inability of the lung to distribute the body fluid. In this case, the triple-jiao as well as the muscular striae are obstructed and the muscles are poorly nourished, so there are polydipsia and emaciation. And direct downward flow of water to the lower-jiao due to disturbance of the water distribution causes the urine to be profuse and sweet in taste. The fire in the lung may arise from the upward attack of the stomach-heat produced by excessive intake of fat or sweet food or indulgence in alcohol, or the upward attack of the heart-fire due to emotional stresses, or the fire from the kidney due to water unable to restrict floating to the lung.

(2) Pathologic change in the middle-jiao

① Excessive stomach-heat: The stomach is where water and food collect, so when heat accumulates and consumes the body fluid in the stomach, polyorexia will occur as a result, which will in turn cause emaciation due to failure of the nutrients to be absorbed and frequent urine. In the case of failure of the large intestine to be moistened due to impairment of the stomach fluid, dry stool will ensue.

In the development of the diabetes involving the middle-jiao, the stomach-heat may go upward to burn the lung, leading to more severe deficiency of the lung-fluid and the ensuing aggravation of the polydipsia. It may aslo run downward to the kidney, leading to more severe consumption of the kidney-fluid and as a result, the diabetes will affect the lower-jiao. In the case the stomach-heat accumulates in the muscles and skin, it may cause carbuncles, sores or furuncles. Therefore, the stomach-heat may be spread to all the three portions of the triple-jiao in the course of diabetes.

② The stomach-fire of the deficiency-type: Consumption of the stomach-yin due to long burning of the stomach-fire may bring about more severe hyperactivity of the fire, which will aggravate the diabetes. In this case, patients may want to eat due to the deficiency or are unable to eat, which will cause abdominal distension and fullness, worsening the disease.

(3) Pathological change in the lower-jiao

This is mainly marked by deficiency and consumption of the kidney and discordance between the heart and the kidney. The kidney dominates water metabolism and stores essence. If fire of deficiency-type involves the kidney, the kidney-qi will be consumed, which may cause disturbance of the steaming function of the kidney and further inability of the kidney to control the water metabolism. As a result, frequent urination with profuse urine will occur. The consumption of the kidney-qi may also lead to inability of the kidney to store essence, giving rise to downward flow of the food essence and the subsequent turbid urine with a sweet taste. The kidney is an organ in which both water and fire exist. Disharmony between the kidney-yin and the kidney-yang and hyperactivity of the kidney-fire due to kidney-yin deficiency are both contributable to occurrence of diabetes.

2) Pathologic influence of the zang-fu organs in the development of diabetes

Man is an organic unity in which the zang-fu organs are closely related to each other physiologically and influence each other pathologically. For example, impairment of the lung-fluid by dryness will cause loss of moistening of the stomach as a result of failure of the lung to distribute body fluid, which will in turn cause deficiency of the kidney-fluid. The deficiency of the kidney-fluid will lead to more severe dryness of the lung due to the upward attack of fire of the deficiency-type. On the other way round, the impairment of the lung-fluid due to dryness may also cause deficiency of the kidney-fluid as a result of the lung unable to distribute the body fluid, which will further bring about the impairment of the stomach-fluid as a result of the fire of deficiency-type from the kidney going upward to attack the stomach. Deficiency of the stomach-fluid will, in turn, lead to more severe consumption of the lung-fluid.

Disorders of different organs of the three types of diabetes may be transmitted to each other. As described above, impairment of the lung- fluid will cause loss of moistening of the stomach and the kidney as a result of failure of the lung to distribute the body fluid; excessive dryness-heat in the spleen and stomach may burn the body fluid, leading to consumption of the kidney-yin and the ensuing hyperactivity of the kidney-fire, which may in turn burn the body-fluid in the lung and stomach. This transmission will eventually lead to coexistence of the lung-dryness, stomach-heat and deficiency of both the spleen and kidney, as a result, polydipsia, polyphagia, polyuria and emaciation are present silmutaneously. Of these affected organs, the kidney is the key organ in the pathological changes of diabetes. Concurrence of the three types of diabetes will be followed in the case of impairment of the kidney due to severe diabetes involving the upper- or the middle-jiao or the deficient kidney-water failing to moisten the lung and stomach.

2.3 The characteristics of pathogenesis

1) Yin-deficiency as the primary cause and dryness-heat as the secondary

Exuberance of the dryness-heat often results from yin-deficiency. But when the dryness-heat is produced, it will cause more severe yin-deficiency. Therefore, yin-deficiency and dryness-heat can be both the cause and result of each other. In other word, the exuberant dryness-heat comes from the yin-deficiency, the more exuberant the dryness-heat is, the more deficient the yin is, and vice versa. Although the diabetes may involve all the five zang-organs and the six fu-organs, it is mainly concerned with the lung, the stomach and the spleen, and the kidney, of which the kidney is the most important. Of the yin-deficiency and dryness-heat, although one aspect may be more obvious, the former always serves as the fundamental cause of the disease and the latter, the secondary. In the clinic, patients always present the manifestations of deficiency while the symptoms of dryness-heat are seen such as polyphagia and polydipsia.

2) Deficiency of both qi and yin and impairment of both yin and yang

22

This disease has a rather long course in which consumption of yin, impairment of yin, or yin-deficiency affecting yang, or even exhaustion of the kidney-yang and depletion of the kidney-qi will occur. In such cases, it will become a critical and severe condition. The old and debility patients with original yang-deficiency or the patients with original deficiency of both yang and qi may present the manifestations of deficiency of both qi and yang at its initial stage, which may cause the decline of the mingmen-fire and further cause failure of the water to be transformed. This kind of diabetes shouldn't be neglected, for it may be very severe in some cases.

3) Deteriorated cases secondary to yin-deficiency and dryness-heat

In the cases of long-standing existence of the disease, erroneous or delayed treatment, the disease may develop variety of deteriorated cases. For example, loss of nourishment of the lung may be followed by pulmonary tuberculosis in a chronic case; and night blindness, nebula and deafness may be secondary to deficiency of the liver-yin and the kidney-yin. As the book *Discussion on Three Types of Diabetes* says: "In diabetics, there often occur deafness, blindness, sores, tinea, acnes, sudamina, etc. , or edema on the face due to upward flow of water. " Diabetes involving the middle-jiao, which is marked by polyphagia and excessive stomach-heat, often leads to stagnation of qi and blood, resulting in carbuncles and sores due to the accumulated toxin producing pus. If cold or cool drugs impair the stomach, the coldness of the middle-jiao will appear while the heat in the upper-jiao remains still, which will cause abdominal fullness. In the case of excessive drinking invading the spleen, the spleen will fail to control the distribution of water, as a result, the water will flow to the muscles and skin to cause edema and distension. In the chapter of Xiaoke Syndrome Category of the book *General Collection for Holy Relief*, it is stated that "those who can eat will have carbuncles of the nape and back at last; those who can not eat will finally develop tympanites marked by abdominal distension. All these diseases are incurable. "

23

Here, desire for food indicates hyperactivity of fire, while inability to eat indicates deficiency of the spleen and stomach. So attentions should be paid to their different pathological basis.

4) The important relationship between the occurrence of diabetes and blood stasis

Blood stasis in diabetics is caused by dryness-heat due to yin-deficiency, consumption and burning of body fluid, abnormality of the peripheral blood circulation and the impeded flow of blood, or by yin-deficiency affecting yang which leads to yang-deficiency, stagnation of cold, and the resultant aggravation of the blood stasis. As is stated in the chapter Occurrence of Thirst in the book *On Blood Stasis*: "The body fluid depends on the kidney-water for its production. Failure gf qi to go up due to obstruction of the blood stasis will therefore obstruct the upward flow of water following the flow of qi, from which thirst occurs. " Blood stasis and diabetes often have both the mutual cause and result. Prolonged interior heat due to yin-deficiency will consume qi and impair yin, leading to deficiency of both qi and yin, while long-standing deficiency of qi and yin will in turn lead to blood stasis as the deficiency-qi is unable to move blood, and obstruction of qi by the blood and disturbed distribution of water, which will finally aggravate the pathological changes in diabetes and the deterioration of the patients' conditions.

To sum up from all this above, the occurrence of diabetes is closely related to the constitutional conditions, excessive intake of the delicious, fat and sweet food, as well as excess of sexual intercourse leading to injury of the kidney, emotional disturbance causing stagnation of the liver-qi, or overuse of pungent , dry and yang-strengthening things(including the cigarettes, alcohol, tonics, etc. , which are considered to be very pungent and very hot in TCM) and so on. But the conspicuous characteristics of the TCM theory is that it stresses the Concept of Wholism, and Syndrome Identification and Corresponding Treatment. In the clinical practice, we should follow what the chapter of Great Treatise on the Valuable Information about Diseases due to Changes of the Six Normal Natural Factors of the book *Plain Questions* says: " Strictly adhere to the pathogenesis to treat a disease so that the flow of qi and blood are promoted and the health restored. "

The above are the discussion in TCM on the causes and pathogenesis of diabetes. Up to now, the mechanism of the naturally-developed diabetes is still not clear enough. According to the affection of the disease, a number of factors may be contributable to the formation of the causes of the disease. Evidently, descriptions of the causes of the disease in TCM are quite reasonable, which are instructive to the routine maintenance and nursing of our health.

Chapter 3 Syndrome Identification and Corresponding Treatment

In the differentiation of symptoms and signs in TCM, diabetes is often classified as three types(upper, middle and lower) according to propriety of polydipsia, polyphagia and polyuria. The diabetes with polydipsia as the main symptoms is referred to as the upper type, that marked by polyphagia is known as the middle-type, and that characterized by polyuria is termed as the lower type. However, these three types often occur in combination, and are in fact the three syndromes of one disease. So they are usually discussed together and collectively called Sanxiao (three types of diabetes), or named Xiaoke in the ancient books. In respect of the causes and pathogenesis of the disease, besides excessive intake of fat and sweet food and intemperance in sexual life, indulgence in alcohol is also an important induction factor, as is pointed out in the 21st chapter Xiaoke Syndrome in the book *Prescriptions Worth One Thousand Gold for Emergencies*: " those with long-standing drinkings will certainly develop diabetes, nothing is hotter than wine. Long drinking continuously will cause exuberant heat in the triple-jiao and the ensuing dryness of the five zang-organs. In this way wood and rock will be dried up, let alone the human beings. " As for the pathogenesis, it is emphasized again in this chapter that "it should be known that the disease is caused by heat due to yin-deficiency", and that " the internal heat will bring about the preference for drinking", etc. This affirmed that heat of the deficiency-type is the main pathologic mechanism of the disease.

In the treatment of diabetes the chapter of Three Types of Xiaoke Syndrome of the book *Medicine Comprenhended* says: "the upper type of diabetes should be treated by moistening the lung assisted by clearing away the stomach-heat; the middle-type should be treated by clearing away the stomach-heat by the aid of nourishing the kidney; and the lower-type should be treated by nourishing the kidney supported by tonifying the lung. " From this we can see that the major therapeutic principle for diabetes is known deeply. Generally speaking, the early stage of the disease is mostly caused by the lung-dryness and the stomach-heat, and belongs to the upper amd middle types; in a longer case, it is mainly marked by the coexistence of both yin-deficiency and dryness-heat; and in a prolonged case, it is characterized by yin-deficiency, deficiency of both qi and yin, and deficiency of both yin and yang, accompanied with blood stasis, and therefore ascribed to the lower type. Although this disease can be treated in accordance with its three types, its treatment must be mainly based on the treatment of the kidney. In chapter Xiaoke Syndrome of the book the *Secret Records in the Stone Chamber*, Chen Shiduo in the Qing Dynasty said: "although diabetes can be divided into the upper, the middle and the lower, it is caused by the kidney-deficiency without exception. Therefore, the treatment should be mainly based on that of kidney without caring about what type it is. " In addition, the complications of diabetes must be prevented and treated in the treatment of the disease, because a variety of complications may occur secondary to yin-deficiency and dryness-heat, the basic pathogenesis of the disease. The following must be mastered in the identification of syndromes of diabetes.

3. 1 Essentials of syndrome identification

3. 1. 1 Differentiation in accordance with the positions

Thirst with desire for excessive drinking and frequent urination with massive urine indicate the upper type of diabetes caused by lung-dryness with dryness-heat as the main pathogenesis.

Polyorexia, polyphagia and thirst indicate the middle type of diabetes caused by stomach-heat with dryness-heat as the main pathogenesis.

The above are excessive in nature.

Frequent urination with massive urine thick and turbid as chyme indicates the lower type of diabetes mainly caused by kidney deficiency, especially the deficiency of the kidney-yin, which is deficient in nature.

3. 1. 2 Differentiation in accordance with deficiency and excess

This disease is marked by deficiency of the vital qi and hyperactivity of the fire in pathogenesis, of which the former is the fundamental and the latter is the fire of the deficiency-type. Excessive fire syndrome may also be seen in diabetics of the middle-aged at the early stage marked by exuberance of pathogenic fire. Deficiency type of the diabetes results mostly from the deficiency of the kidney-yin. These two different syndromes must be differentiated in the clinic with great care.

1) Excessive syndrome

This is marked by extreme thirst with profuse drinking, polyorexia, dysphoria, dry stool, frequent or dark urine, emaciation, yellow tongue coating and rapid pulse.

2) Deficiency syndrome

This is characterized by feverish sensation over the palms, soles and chest with restlessness, dark complexion, dry and withered helix, flushed face, red lips, night sweating, poor appetite, emaciation, dark urine or incontinence of urine which is as thick as chyme with a sweet taste of bran, red tongue with little coating, weak, thready and rapid or weak, floating and hollow pulse.

While the excess or deficiency is differentiated, whether there is fire or not should be differentiat at the same time. Diabetes may be caused by either depletion of water or deficiency of fire. In the case of decline of the mingmen-fire, yang will fail to transform and distribute the body fluid. As a result, the water will flow downwards directly to the bladder and fail to go upward, leading to polyuria. This is a syndrome of deficiency of the genuine yang and depletion of fire in the lower-jiao and used to be very severe because of both yin and yang are exhausted.

3) Differentiation of the mild, serious and critical cases: Gao Gufeng of the Qing Dynasty said in the chapter Xiaoke Syndrome of his book *Treatise on the Duties for Medical Professionals*: "in the three types of diabetes, the upper and the middle types can be cured, but the lower type is difficult to cure; urinating as much as drinking can be cured, but urinating twice as much as drinking cannot be cured." Dai Yuanli of the Yuan Dynasty wrote, in the chapter Three Types of Xiaoke Syndrome of his book *The Important Knack of Diagnosis and Treatment*, "In the long term of the diabetes urine with no stink but sweet taste rolling in the urinal indicates a critical condition, and that spilling at the side of the urinal like candle tears indicates the unconsolidation of the essence-qi and the exhaustion of the kidney-essence.

In protracted diabetes, transmission and accompanying diseases often develops. For example, lingering upper type of the diabetes may cause impairment of yin and deficiency of qi, leading to the transmission from the upper-type to the middle and lower types; long term existence of the middle-type, as a result of the fire burning the lung and the kidney, may spread to the upper and the lower, or may consume the yin-fluid of the spleen and stomach; and protracted lower type may cause yin-deficiency affecting yang or impairment of both yin and yang; etc.

3. 2 Essentials of treatment

3. 2. 1 The mastery of the therapeutic principle

Pathogeneses of diabetes are fundamentally the yin-deficiency and the dryness-heat, which should be treated by nourishing yin and moistening the dryness incombination. This is performed by moistening the lung in the case of the upper type, clearing away heat from the stomach in the case of the middle type and nourishing the kidney in the case of the lower type. If yin affects yang in a chronic case, tonifying both yin and yang should be adopted, and if blood stasis is complicated, activating blood flow to remove blood stasis should be employed simultaneously.

3. 2. 2 The mastery of therapeutic law

1) Applying more tonics and less purgatives of cool or cold nature

Diabetes is a chronic disease which is marked by excessive discharge of fluid and essence through urination and the ensuing deficiency of the vital-qi in a prolonged case. So, it should be mainly treated with tonics. Formulas of extremely cold or cool such as Da Chengqi Tang(Major Decoction for Promoting Flow of Qi in the Large Intestine) should not be used carelessly. When it is used to treat disorder of the heart and the lung, its dose should be small, while if it is used to treat disorders of the liver and kidney, its dose may be larger. In the treatment of the upper and middle types of diabetes, reducing fire should be employed but can not be too impatiently in order to avoid the cold or cool drugs impairing the stomach. If this is not followed, cold in the middle-jiao will be produced while the heat in the upper is not expelled, which may cause abdominal distension in a chronic case.

2) Treating the new and old diseases with different methods

In the initial stage the treatment should be aimed at the heart and the lung and in the chronic cases at the spleen and the kidney. For the upper type, clearing fire from the lung should be employed at the early stage, while in a prolonged condition, nourishing yin and moistening dryness or supplementing qi should be adopted. For the middle type, the treatment should be directed at clearing away fire from the stomach at the early stage and at tonifying the spleen to control the essence(qi) at the later. For the lower type, the treatment should be to nourish yin to clear away heat at the early stage and to tonify both yin and yang because of the yin-deficiency affecting yang at the later. All the three types of diabetes are closely related to the kidney,

30

so treatment of the kidney forms the basis of all the other treatments.

3) Treating the three types of diabetes differently with the treatment of the kidney as its basis

One of the key to the treatment of diabetes is to master the "three methods of treating the kidney" flexibly. Usually, the treatment should be to nourish water to clear away heat for cases with exuberance of fire due to yin-deficiency. For those with severe depletion of the yin-essence in the chronic cases, the treatment should be supported by tonifying the essence and consolidating the lower orificies. For those with failure of qi to control essence due to yin-deficiency affecting yang, the treatment should be assisted by strengthening water and supplementing qi. Warming the yang in the lower should be applied to ascend and control water for the old patients with decline of ming-men-fire and inability of qi to tranform the water. In the cases of floating of the fire of deficiency-type, inducing the fire to go downwards should be adopted in the treatment.

3. 2. 3 Preventing and treating complications

Treatment of diabetes should be centred on the prevention and treatment of the complications. For details, see a special chapter of this book.

3. 3 Syndromes identification and corresponding treatment

3. 3. 1 Diagnosis and treatment according to the different types of diabetes

Doctors throughout ages have been diagnosing and treating the disease based on the three types of the disease. Usually, the upper type of diabetes is marked by polydipsia, the middle-type by polyphagia and the lower type by polyuria. This is used as the sign to perform syndromes identification and corresponding treatment.

1) The upper type of diabetes marked by impairment of the body fluid due to lung-heat

Manifestations: polydipsia, dry tongue and mouth, frequent urination with profuse urine, polyphagia, red tongue tip and border,thin and yellow coating, full and rapid pulse.

Analysis: As the lung is an organ with purifying and descending function, excessive heat in the lung will cause consumption of body fluid, leading to dry mouth and tongue, and polydipsia. The lung dominates the regulation of the distribution of water. Dryness-heat impairing the lung will result in the failure of the water to be transformed into the body fluid and its downward flow to cause frequent urination with much urine. Dryness-heat in the stomach is responsible for polyphagia. And red tongue tip and border, thin and yellow coating, and full and rapid pulse all indicate dryness-heat in the lung. In addition, red tongue tip also indicates the heart-fire.

Therapeutic method: Clearing away heat and moistening the lung, promoting the production of the body fluid to quench thirst.

Prescription: Xiaoke Fang (Prescription for Treating Diabetes, from *Danxi's Experiential Therapy*) with modification. In this recipe, Hua Fen (Radix Trichosanthis) is used in a high dose to clear away heat and promote the production of body fluid to quench thirst; Huang Lian (Rhizoma Coptidis), as an adjunvant drug, to clear away heat and purge fire, and as a bitter drug, to clearing away the heat from the heart in a particular so as to lower down the heart-fire and avoid the further impairment of the lung; Sheng Di (Radix Rehmanniae), Ou Zhi (juice of Lotus), etc. , to nourish yin and moisten dryness. Besides, Ge Gen (Radix Puerariae) and Mai Dong (Radix Ophiopogonis) can be added to strengthen the function of nourishing yin and promoting the production of the body fluid to quench thirst.

For cases with full, rapid but forceless pulse, polydipsia and frequent urination due to deficiency of both qi and yin of the lung and the kidney, Erdong Tang (Decoction of Radix Asparagi and Radix Ophiopogonis, from *Medical Comprehended*) with modifications can be adopted as an alternative. In this formula, Ren Shen (Radix Ginseng) is used to supplement qi and promote the production of body fluid, Tian Dong (Radix Asparagi), Mai Dong (Radix Ophiopogonis) and Hua Fen (Radix Trichosanthis) to nourish yin and promote the production of body fluid to quench thirst, and Huang Qin (Radix Scutellariae) and Zhi Mu (Rhizoma Anemarrhenae) to purge fire to preserve yin.

For cases with yellow and dry tongue coating, rapid and large pulse, dysphoria, polydipsia, or accompanied with polyphagia and dry stool, which indicate heat in both the lung and the stomach impairing qi and yin, Baihu Jia Renshen Tang (White Tiger Decoction with Ginseng, from *Synopsis of Prescriptions of the Golden Chamber*) can be employed to clear away heat from the lung and the stomach, promote the production of body fluid and supplement qi so that the body fluid can be regenerated while the heat is removed. As the exuberant heat in the lung and stomach consumes qi and yin, Ren Shen (Radix Ginseng) is added to the formula to supplement qi, promote the production of body fluid and nourish yin.

The disorders of the heart and lung in the upper type of diabetes induce frquently the hyperactivity of the stomach-fire and the kidney-fire, resulting in combination of the upper type with the middle type, or that of the upper type with the lower type. At this time, if the upper type is still dominant, the treatment should be still aimed at the treatment of the lung, assisted by clearing away the stomach-heat and nourishing the stomach-yin, and purging fire and nourishing the kidney.

2) The middle-type of diabetes marked by exuberance of the stomach-fire

Manifestations: polyphagia, polydipsia, emaciation, dry stool, frequent urination with sweet urine, dry and yellow tongue coating, slippery, solid and forceful pulse.

Analysis: The stomach is in charge of receiving food. Hyperactivity of the stomach-fire will increase the digestive function of the stomach, from which polyphagia results. Dryness-heat in the gastrointesti-

33

nal tract impairs the body fluid, so there is polydipsia, the manifestation of self-helping. Consumption of the body fluid and blood due to exuberant heat in the yangming meridian causes inability of the muscles to be nourished and the ensuing emaciation. The insufficient stomach-fluid failing to moisten the large intestine is responsible for dry stool. And hyperactivity of the kidney-yang due to kidney-yin deficiency and unconsolidation of the kidney-qi lead to polyuria. The yellow tongue coating and slippery, solid and forceful pulse indicate exuberance of the stomach-fire.

Therapeutic method: Purging the stomach-fire, nourishing yin and preserving the body fluid.

Prescription: Yunu Jian (Gypsum Decoction, from *Jingyue's Complete Medical Books*) with Huang Lian (Rhizoma Coptidis) and Zhi Zi (Fructus Gardeniae) added.

In this formula, Sheng Shi Gao (Gypsum Fibrosum) and Zhi Mu (Rhizoma Anemarrhenae) are used to clear away heat from the lung and the stomach; Sheng Di (Radix Rehmanniae) and Mai Dong (Radix Ophiopogonis) to nourish the lung-yin and the stomach-yin; Huang Lian (Rhizoma Coptidis) and Zhi Zi (Fructus Gardeniae) to clear away heat and purge fire; and Niu Xi (Radix Achyranthis Bidentatae) to induce the heat to flow downwards.

In the case of constipation, Zengye Chengqi Tang (Purgative Decoction for Increasing Fluid and Sustaining Qi, from *Treatise on Differentiation and Treatment of Epidemic Febrile Diseases*) can be used to moisten dryness and remove obstruction from the fu-organs, and jointly, Tiaowei Chengqi Tang (Purgative Decoction for Coordination the Function of the Stomach) can be used to remove the stagnated fire by promoting the bowel movement to preserve the stomach-fluid. When the bowel is relaxd, the above formula should be applied.

3) The lower-type of diabetes marked by deficiency of the kidney-yin and deficiency of both yin and yang

(1) Deficiency of the kidney-yin

34

Manifestations: Frequent urination with much urine as turbid as chyme or with a sweet taste, polydipsia, soreness and weakness of th loins and knees, dry mouth lips, feverish sensation over the palms, soles and chest, red tongue, deep, thready and rapid pulse.

Analysis: The deficient kidney failing to control urination leads to polyuria; unconsolidation of the kidney-qi causes the food essence to flow downward, resulting in turbid urine with a sweet taste; failure of the feverish sensation and dysphoria leads to interior heat and the ensuing polydipsia; kidney- deficiency and the resultant loss of nourishment of the loins lead to soreness and weakness of the loins and knees. Dry mouth and lips, feverish sensation over the palms, soles and chest, red tongue and deep, thready and rapid pulse signify deficiency of the kidney-yin and the subsequent hyperativity of fire.

Therapeutic method: Nourishing yin and consolidating the kidney.

Prescription: Liuwei Dihuang Wan (Bolus of Six Drugs Including Rehmannia Root, from *Key to Therapeutics of Children's Diseases*), or Zuogui Yin (Drink for Tonifying the Kidney-yin, from *Jingyue's Complete Medical Books*).

The doses of Shan Yao (Rhizoma Dioscoreae) and Shan Yu Rou (Fructus Corni) in Zuogui Yin should be larger, for Shan Yao functions to benifit the spleen-yin to control the food essence, and assisted by Shan Yu Rou, to consolidate the kidney to prevent food essence from flowing downwards and strengthen the storing function of the kidney. Shu Di (Radix Rehmanniae Praeparata) and Gou Qi Zi (Fructus Lycii) are used to tonify the kidney and supplement the fluid, and Fu Ling (Poria) and Gan Cao (Radix Glycyrrhizae) to nourish yin and clear away heat. Combined use of the above drugs has the function of tonifying the kidney, supplementing essence and strengthening the consolidating function of the kidney.

For cases with hyperactivity of fire due to yin-deficiency marked by restlessness, insomnia, nocturnal emission, red tongue and thready rapid pulse, Huang Bai (Cortex Phellodendri), Zhi Mu (Rhi-

35

zoma Anemarrhenae), Long Gu(Os Draconis), Mu Li(Concha Ostreae) and Gui Ban(Plastrum Testudinis) can be added to the above formula to nourish yin and clear away heat, arresting emission and checking the hyperactive yang.

For cases with profuse turbid urine, Yi Zhi Ren(Fructus Alpiniae Oxyphyllae), Sang Piao Xiao(Ootheca Mantidis), Wu Wei Zi(Fructus Schisandrae) and Can Jian(Coccum Bombycis),etc. can be added to the above formula to tonify the kidney, reduce urine, strengthen the consolidating effect of the kidney and astringe the emission.

For cases with deficiency of both qi and yin marked by lassitude, shortness of breath and light red tongue, the above formula can be used in combination with Shengmai San(Pulse Activating Powder, from *Discussion on the Differentiation of Endogenous and Exogenous Diseases*) to tonify the lung-qi and the kidney-qi. For cases with qi deficiency, Dang Shen(Radix Codonopsis Pilosulae) , Huang Qi(Radix Astragali seu Hedysari),etc. should be added to supplement qi.

(2) Deficiency of both yin and yang

Manifestations: Frequent urination with clear water-like or turbidchyme-like urine, thirst but drinking little, or urinating twice as much as drinking, dark, lustreless and withered face, parched and dry helix, soreness and weakness of the loins and knees, aversion to cold, cold limbs, edema or oliguria, or diarrhea at dawn, impotence, premature ejaculation, pale tongue with white and slippery coating,deep thready but forceless pulse.

Analysis: Long deficiency of the kidney-yin affecting yang leads to decline of the reserving function of the kidney, sinking of the kidney-qi, and dysfunction of the kidney-yang, causing the clear water-like urine; sinking of the kidney-qi is responsible for the turbid chyme-like urine; decline of the mingmen-fire and deficiency of the kidney-water leads to failure of the fire to steam upward and that of the water to go upward, causing lung-dryness marked by thirst which is accompanied with little drinking because the fire is not so exuber-

36

ant; the deficient kidney-qi failing to control the urine gives rise to frequent urination or even urinating twice as much as drinking; downward flow of the food essence with the urine leads to its failure to nourish the whole body and inability of the residual fluid to be excreted, causing dark, lustreless and withered face; the kidney is in charge of bones and opens into the ears, and the waist houses the kidney, so the kideny deficiency causes parched and dry helix, soreness and weakness of the loins and knees; decline of the mingmen-fire and the ensuing failure of yang to perform its warming effect lead to relaxation of the penis and unsolidation of the kidney essence, causing aversion to cold, cold limbs, impotence, and premature ejaculation. Pale tongue with whitish coating and deep thready but forceless pulse also indicate deficiency of both yin and yang.

Therapeutic method: Warming up yang, nourishing yin and consolidating the reserving function of the kidney.

Prescription: Jinkui Shengqi Wan (Bolus of Golden Chamber for Tonifying the Kidney-Qi, from *Synopsis of the Prescriptions of the Golden Chamber*).

In this recipe, Fu Zi (Radix Aconiti) and Rou Gui (Cortex Cinnamomi) are used to warm up the kidney-yang; Shu Di Huang (Radix Rehmanniae Praeparata), Shan Yao (Rhizoma Dioscoreae), Shan Yu Rou (Fructus Corni), Dan Pi (Cortex Moutan Radicis), Ze Xie (Rhizoma Alismatis) and Fu Ling (Poria) to tonify the kidney-essence to lay the basis for the ascending of the body fluid. For cases with deficiency of yin, yang, qi and blood, Lurong Wan (Bolus of Pilose and Deer Horn, from *Prescriptions Assigned to the Three Categories of Pathogenic Factors of Diseases*) should be applied as an alternative. To the above two formulas, Fu Pen Zi (Fructus Rubi), Sang Piao Xiao (Ootheca Mantis) and Jin Ying Zi (Rosae Laevigatae) can be added.

To sum up, of the three types of diabetes, the lower type is the most serious. Diabetes is a deficient disease in nature with pathologic change of the kidney as the centre and is mostly caused by debility in the aged, prolonged diseases, congenital deficiency and intemperance in sexual life. The above introduced are the basic methods of syndrome identification for diabetes, which is mainly manifested by polydipsia, polyphagia, polyuria and emaciation. As a chronic disease, occurrence of diabetes is mostly related to excessive intake of fat and delicious food, emotional disturbance or excessive sexual activity, or hereditary factors in some cases. Hyperactivity of fire due to yin-deficiency is the fundamental pathogenesis of the disease and usually involves the lung, the stomach and the kidney. With the development of the disease, impairment of both qi and yin, deficiency of both yin and yang, or other pathologic changes may occur. Of the secondary conditions, carbuncles, sores and furuncles are the most commonly encountered. In treatment tonifying the kidney to strengthen the basis of the life should, therefore, be used according to the patients' condition besides nourishing yin to treat the fundamental causes and clearing away heat to treat the secondary causes. Clearing away the lung-heat and moistening dryness or supplementing qi and nourishing yin in the chronic case can be used for the upper type of diabetes; purging the pathogenic fire and clearing away the lung-heat or strengthening the spleen and controlling essence in the chronic case for the middle type; and nourishing the kidney to reduce the hyperactive fire or tonifying the kidney to consolidate the kidney esesence in the chronic case for the lower type. In the case of failure of qi to transform water due to yin-deficiency affecting yang, tonifying the essence and warming and supporting yang should be adopted to transform water. In any type of the diabetes, tonifying the kidney should be noticed when the kidney is involved, and if the spleen deficiency occurs in the protracted case, strengthening the spleen to control essence should be employed to restore the coordination between the heart and the kidney.

3. 3. 2 Diagnosis and treatment in accordance with pathologic

changes of the zang-fu organs

TCM is a discipline with the theory of zang-fu as its core, syndrome identification and corresponding treatment as its principle, and the concept of wholism as its guiding ideology. For this reason, diabetes can be diagnosed and treated in accordance with the zang-fu theory besides the three types of diabetes.

1) Disorders of the heart

The heart controls both blood circulation and mental activities. Therefore, disorders of the heart are mainly manifested as disturbed blood circulation and abnormal mental activities. Clinically, disorders of the heart can be divided into two groups, the deficient and the excessive.

(1) Deficient syndromes of the heart

① Deficiency of the heart-yin:

Main manifestations: Palpitation, sleeplessness or insomnia, amnesia, red tongue with little coating or red and dry tongue tip, thready rapid pulse. This kind of palpitation is usually accompanied with dysphoria and throbbing, and the sleeplessness, with dream-disturbed sleep.

Therapeutic method: Nourishing yin, tonifying the heart and tranquilizing the mind.

Prescription: Tianwang Buxin Dan (Cardiotonic Pill, from Secret Prescriptions for Keeping Health), Siwu Tang (Decoction of Four Ingredients, from Prescriptions of People's Welfare Pharmacy), and so like.

For cases with severe sleeplessness, insomnia and amnesia, add Nu Zhen Zi (Fructus Ligustri Lucidi) 10g and Shou Wu Teng (Caulis Polygoni Multiflori) 20g; for cases with severe palpitation, add Shi Chang Pu (Rhizoma Acori Graminei) 10g and Yuan Zhi (Radix Polygalae) 10g; and for cases with dream-disturbed sleep, add Bai Wei (Radix Cynanchi Atrati) 10g.

② Deficiency of the heart-yang:

39

Main manifestations: Palpitation, shortness of breath, chest stuffiness, precordial pain, pale tongue, weak or knotted and intermittent pulse. Palpitation of this type is marked by an empty feeling in the heart with throbbing which is more serious on exertion; the shortness of breath usually occurs paroxysmally and will also be aggravated on exertion; the precordial pain has a sudden onset, mostly accompanied with cold limbs, extremely rapid and scattered pulse, or even dark, lustreless and purplish hands, feet, lips and nose, or with pale complexion, aversion to cold and spontaneous sweating.

Therapeutic method: Warming up the heart-yang and invigorating the heart-qi.

Prescription: Guizhi Jia Fuzi Tang (Cinnamon Twig and Aconite Decoction, from *Treatise on Febrile Diseases*) or Yangxin Tang (Decoction for Tonifying the Heart, from *Standards of Diagnosis and Treatment*).

In the above formulas, Gui Zhi functions to promote flow of the heart-yang. In the case of palpitation with a knotted and intermittent pulse, Gui Zhi 20g can be applied. If hypoactivity of the chest-yang and obstruction of phlegm in the chest are also present, Xie Bai (Bulbus Allii Macrostemi) can be added to promote the flow of yang-qi and remove obstruction. Combined use of Xie Bai and Gua Lou (Fructus Trichosanthis) can be effective for angina pectoris, like the effect of Gualou Xiebai Banxia Tang (Decoction of Trichosanthes, Allium and Pinellia). In addition, Gua Lou has the effect of relieving chest distension and dissolving phlegm. Together with Bei Mu (Bulbus Fritillariae) and Xing Ren (Semen Armeniacae Amarum), it can ventilate the lung and dissolve phlegm, and together with Zhi Shi (Fructus Aurantii Imaturus) and Ban Xia (Rhizoma Pinelliae), it can treat chest fullness and shortness of breath.

③ Deficiency of the heart-qi:

Qi belongs to yang and blood belongs to yin. Therefore, deficiency of the heart-yang is always complicated by deficiency of the heart-qi, and deficiency of the heart-yin is always accompanied with deficiency of the heart-blood. However, deficiency of the heart-yang is more serious than that of the heart-qi. So, in the treatment of deficiency of the heart-yang, in addition to tonifying the heart-yang, invigorating qi should also be adopted. Generally speaking, drugs with the action of invigorating qi exert a tonic effect on the human body through strengthening the physiologic function and improving the strength. Thus such qi-tonics as Huang Qi (Radix Astragalis seu Hedysari), Ren Shen(Radix Ginseng), Dang Shen(Radix Codonopsis Pilosulae), etc. should be employed when deficiency of the heart-qi occurs. In the case of deficiency of both the heart-yang and the heart-yin, Zhigancao Tang (Decoction of Prapared Licorice, from *Treatise on Febrile Diseases*)should be selected to tonify both the heart-yin and the heart-yang. For the case with consumption of both qi and blood, Shiquan Dabu Tang(Bolus of Ten Powerful Tonics, from *Prescriptions of People's Welfare Pharmacy*) should be administered to tonify both qi and blood. If knotted and intermittent pulse presents as a result of deficiency of the heart-qi, the dosage of Gui Zhi(Ramulus Cinnamomi) should be increased.

(2) Excessive syndromes of the heart

① Hyperactivity of the heart-fire:

Main manifestations: Red tongue tip, or dysphoria, palpitation, insomnia, erosion of the tongue and mouth, scanty and dark urine, rapid pulse.

The tongue is the sprout of the heart which is interior-exteriorly related to the small intestines. So, the exuberance of the heart-fire causes red tongue tip, erosions of the tongue and mouth, dysphoria and palpitation. Downward transmission of the exuberant heart-fire to the small intestine is responsible for the dark and scanty urine.

Therapeutic method: Purging the heart-fire.

Prescription: Daochi San(Powde for Treating Dark Urine, from *Key to Therapeutics of Children's Diseases*).

To the formula, Huang Lian(Rhizoma Coptidis) 6 — 10g, Huang Qin(Radix Scutellariae) 10g and Lian Qiao(Frcutus Forsythiae) 6g can be added deliberately. For cases with erosions of the tongue and mouth, Sheng Pu Huang(Pollen Typhae) 10g, Sheng Ma(Rhizoma Cimicifugae) 6g and Pu Gong Ying(Herba Taraxaci) 30g are to be added.

If the exuberance of the heart-fire arises from the yin-deficiency, which is marked by restlessness, insomnia, erosion of the tongue, red tongue, and thready rapid pulse, it indicates a deficient syndrome, which should be treated by nourishing yin and clearing away heat from the heart with Tianwang Buxin Dan(Cardiotonic Pill) plus Huang Lian(Rhizoma Coptidis), Zhi Zi(Fructus Gardeniae), etc.

For cases with exuberance of fire due to yin-deficiency, marked by feverish sensation over the palms, soles and chest, nocturnal emission and soreness of the loins, Zhibai Dihuang Wang(Rehamnnia Root Decoction with Anemarrha and Phellodendron) can be used with modifications to nourish yin and reduce fire.

② Obstruction of the heart blood:

Main manifestations: Palpitation or severe palpitation, stuffiness or stabbing pain over the chest and precordial region, which radiates to the shoulders and the medial side of the arms and happens on and off, dark red tongue tip or dotted with ecchymosis, thready and uneven or knotted and intermittent pulse; or in severe cases, sudden pain in the chest and precordial region, purplish lips, cold limbs, unconsciousness, feeble and indistinct pulse.

This syndrome is usually caused by deficiency of the heart-qi or deficiency of the heart-yang, which leads to loss of warmth and activation of vessels, stagnation of qi in the vessels and the ensuing blood stasis and disturbance of blood flow in the vessels.

Therapeutic method: Activating blood flow, removing obstructions in the collaterals and the blood stasis.

Prescription: Xuefu Zhuyu Tang(Decoction for Removing Blood

42

Stasis in the Chest, from Corrections on the Errors of Medical Works), Guanxin Erhao (Prescription No. 2 for CHD),etc.

Drugs activating the blood flow , such as Dan Shen(Radix Salviae Miltiorrhizae), Chi Shao (Radix Paeoniae Rubra), Chuan Xiong (Rhizoma Ligustici Chuanxiong), Hong Hua (Flos Carthami), Pu Huang(Pollen Typhae), Tao Ren (Semen Persicae) and Dang Gui (Radix Angelicae Sinensis) can all be added to the above formulas according to the patients' conditions, and both the fundamental and secondary causes of the disease should be treated at the same time.

(3) Combined syndromes

① Deficiency of both the heart and the spleen:

Main manifestations: Sallow complexion, poor appetite, lassitude, shortness of breath, listlessness, palpitation, amnesia, insomnia with dream- disturbed sleep, irregular menstruation in females, thready and weak pulse,pale tongue with whitish coating.

The heart dominates the blood and blood vessles, and the spleen is related to anxiety. Over anxiety,therefore,impairs both the heart and the spleen, leading to deficiency of the yin-blood and dysfunction of the spleen. As a result of the deficient blood failing to nourish the heart and go upward to nourish the face and the brain, the above symptoms ensue.

Therapeutic method: Tonifying the heart-blood, supplementing qi and tranquilizing the mind.

Prescription: Guipi Tang (Decoction for Invigorating the Spleen and Nourishing the Heart, from *Prescriptions for Benovalence*) with modification, to which Ren Shen(Radix Ginseng),Huang Qi(Radix Astragali seu Hedysari), Bai Zhu(Rhizoma Atractylodis Macrocephalae), Dang Gui (Radix Angelicae Sinensis), Gui Yuan Rou(Arillus Longan),Gan Cao(Radix Glycyrrhizae), etc. , can be added to or reduced from the formula in accordance with the patients' conditions.

② Breakdown of the normal physiologic coordination between the heart and the kidney:

43

Main manifestations: Dysphoria, insomnia, palpitation, amnesia, dizziness and vertigo, dry throat, tinnitus, soreness and weakness of the loins and knees, nocturnal emission, frequent urination at night, hectic fever, night sweat, weak and rapid pulse, red tongue without coating.

Disturbance of the physiologic relation between the heart-yang and the kidney-yin, deficiency of the kidney-yin or abnormal activity of the heart-yang can all lead to breakdown of the harmonious connections between the heart and the kidney, which is known as breakdown of the normal physiologic coordination between the heart and the kidney. Physiologically, the heart, which corresponds to fire in the five elements and stores spirit, and the kidney, which corresponds to water in the five elements and stores essence, are both supplementary to each other and restrict each other, thereby maintaining their normal physiological functions. To be exact, the genuine yang of the kidney ascends to warm up the heart-yang so that the heart-fire can go down to the kidney to prevent the overflow of the kidney-water and assist the genuine yang, on the other hand, the kidney-water restricts the heart-fire so that the heart-fire would not be too excessive and the heart-yin is supplemented. This relation is called mutual assistance between the water and fire. In diabetics, exuberance of fire due to yin-deficiency and deficiency of the kidney-yin failing to restrict the heart-fire will cause hyperactivity of the heart-fire, leading to breakdown of the normal physiologic coordination between the heart and the kidney.

Therapeutic method: Restoring the coordination between the heart and the kidney.

Prescription: Huanglian Ejiao Tang (Decoction of Coptis and Colla Corii Asini, from *Treatise on Febrile Diseases*), Jiaotai Wan (Pill for Restoring the Normal Coordination between the Heart and the Kidney, from *Han's Book on Medicine*) or the other formulas of this kind. Of the ingredients, Huang Lian (Rhizoma Coptidis), Huang Qin

44

(Radix Scutellariae), Lian Zi Xin (Plumula Nelumbinis), Lian Qiao Xin (Plumula Forsythiae) and Dan Zhu Ye (Herba Lophatheri) functions to clear away heat from the heart and restore the coordination between the heart and the kidney.

2) Disorders of the lung

The lung is in charge of qi and respiration. Therefore, disorders of the lung are mainly manifested as the disturbance of the ascending, descending, in-going and out-going of qi. Affection of exogenous pathogens or tuberculosis will involve the lung first, causing the internal impairment of the lung. Disorders of the lung can also be divided into two groups, the deficient and the excessive.

(1) Deficient syndromes of the lung

① Deficiency of the lung-yin and exuberance of dryness-heat:

Main manifestations: The type of loss of moistening of the lung due to the attack of pathogenic dryness is marked by dry cough with little and sticky sputum, or blood-tingled sputum, dry mouth, nose, lips, dry, itching and sore throat, or accompanied with the manifestations of exterior syndrome such as slight aversion to cold, fever and stuffy nose, red tongue tip and border with thin whitish or thin yellowish coating, floating rapid or wiry, thready and rapid pulse. The type of scorching of deficienct fire in the interior due to deficiency of the lung-yin is marked by dry cough with little or blood-stained sputum, hoarsenss, red cheeks in the afternoon, hective fever, night sweating, emaciation, red tongue tip with little coating, thready rapid pulse.

Therapeutic method: Clearing away heat from the lung and moistening the dryness, nourishing yin to moisten the lung.

Prescription: Sang Xing Tang (Decoction of Mulberry Leaf and Apricot Kernel, from *Treatise on Differentiation and Treatment of Epidemic Febrile Diseases*), Qingzao Jiufei Tang (Decoction for Relieving Dryness of the Lung, from *Principle and Prohibition for Medical Profession*), Baihe Gujin Tang (Lily Decoction for Strengthening the Lung, from

45

Collection of Prescriptions with Notes), Shashen Maidong Tang(Decoction of Glehnia and Ophiopogon, from *Treatise on Differentiation of Epidemic Febrile Diseases*), etc.

The ingredients of the above formulas should be adopted deliberately according to patients' conditions. For cases with severe thirst, doses of Tian Hua Fen(Radix Trichosanthis) and Ge Fen(Concha Meretricis) can be increased to 30g respectively. As diabetics often suffer from pulmonary tuberculosis and the lung-heat impairing the lung-yin often occurs in the early stage of diabetes, they can be diagnosed and treated based on the above.

② Deficiency of the Lung-qi:

Main manifestations: Cough with shortness of breath, lassitude, disinclination to talk, low voice, lustreless face, aversion to wind and cold, or spontaneous sweating, pale tongue with whitish coating, weak pulse.

The lung is where all the vessles of the body converge and functions to assist the heart in the circulation of blood. Disturbance of the lung-qi and the ensuing impeded flow of the heart blood cause chest fullness and epistaxis; and inability of the lung-qi to disperse leads to cough and dyspea.

Therapeutic method: Supplementing the lung-qi.

Prescription: Bufei Tang(Decoction for Tonifying the Lung, from *Permanent Effective Prescriptions*), or the other formulas of this kind.

Dang Shen(Radix Codonopsis), or Tai Zi Shen(Radix Pseudostellariae), Huang Qi(Radix Astragali seu Hedysari), Ren Shen(Radix Ginseng), Wu Wei Zi(Fructus Schisandrae), Shan Yao(Rhizoma Dioscoreae), Shu Di(Radix Rehmanniae Praeparata) can be adopted.

(2) The excessive syndrome

The excessive syndrome of the lung is mainly marked by exuberance of the lung-heat, which can be treated with the recipe for lung-dryness and exuberance of fire to which Sang Bai Pi(Cortex Mori

Radicis), Ge Fen (Powder of Concha Meretricis seu Cyslinae), Huang Qin(Radix Scutellariae), etc. are to be added.

(3) Combined syndromes

① Deficiency of both the Lung-yin and the kidney-yin:

Main manifestations: Cough which is severe at night, little sputum or blood-stained sputum, dry mouth and throat, soreness and weakness of the loins and knees, shortness of breath on mild exertion, bone-heat and hective fever, night sweating, red cheeks, nocturnal emission, irregular menstruation in females, red tongue with little coating, thready and rapid pulse.

Therapeutic method: Nourishing the kidney and tonifying the lung.

Prescription: Combined Liuwei Dihuang Wan(Bolus of Six Drugs Including Rehmannia Root) and Shengmai San(Pulse-Activiting Powder) or the like. Ingredients of the recipe include Sha Shen(Radix Adenophorae Strictae), Mai Dong(Radix Ophiopogonis), Tian Dong (Radix Asparagi), Ming Dang Shen (Radix Codonopsis), Shi Hu (Herba Dendrobii), Yu Zhu(Rhizoma Polygonati Odorati) and Bai He(Bulbus Lilii) which function to nourish yin and moisten the lung; and Gou Qi Zi(Fructus Lycii), Nu Zhen Zi(Fructus Ligustri Lucidi), Han Lian Cao (Herba Ecliptae), Shan Yao (Rhizoma Dioscoreae), Shan Yu Rou (Fructus Corni) and Di Huang (Radix Rehmanniae) which function to nourish the kidney.

② The liver-fire attacking the lung:

Main manifestations: Pain in the chest and hypochondrium, irritability, dizziness, red eyes, dry mouth with a bitter taste, paroxysmal cough, or even haemetemesis, red tongue with thin and yellowish coating, wiry and rapid pulse.

Therapeutic method: Clearing away heat from the liver and purging fire from the lung.

Prescription: Daige San(Powder of the Natural Indigo and Clam Shell) and Xiebai San(Powder for Expelling Lung-Heat, from *Key to*

Therapeutics of Children's Diseases) in combination.

Besides, Di Gu Pi (Cortex Lycii Radicis), Huang Qin (Radix Scutellariae), Sang Bai Pi (Cortex Mori Radicis), Bei Mu (Bulbus Fritillariae), Long Dan Cao (Radix Gentianae), Shan Zhi (Fructus Gardeniae), Qing Dai (Indigo Naturalis), etc., can be selected deliberately.

The lung is a delicate organ which is pure and located in the upper. Therefore, formulas for treating disorders of the lung are usually those mild in action and light in weight instead of those heavy in weight and turbid in nature. Just as Wu Jutong said: "Drugs used to treat disorder of the upper-jiao should be as light as feathers, otherwise they will not act on the lung." As a delicate organ, the lung is easily impaired by both pathogenic cold and pathogenic heat, and has a property of desiring for moistening and aversing to dryness, for dryness will induce the lung-qi to go upward to cause cough and asthma, and moistening the lung can help the lung-qi to descend. So drugs pungent, bland or sweet with moistening effect are most suitable for the treatment of the lung disorders and serve as the main drugs for the treatment of diabetes. As for the common accompanying syndromes, the treatment should be based on the severity of the accompanying symptoms. When the main symptoms are relieved, the diabetes should be still treated in accordance with the results of syndrome identification or the types of diabetes according to the patients' conditions.

3) Disorders of the spleen

The spleen is interior-exteriorly related to the stomach, functions to transform and transport foodstuff and control the flow of blood, while the stomach functions to receive and primarily digests the food. Physiologically, the ascending property of the spleen and the descending property of the stomach, and the dryness of the stomach and the moistening of the spleen, assist each other, so that they functions coorperatively to fulfil the digestion, absorption and distribution of

48

the food. In diabetics the exuberant stomach-heat will lead to extremely increased digesting function of the stomach, causing polyphagia and polydipsia. In some cases, impairment of both the spleen and stomach due to improper diet such as excessive intake of raw and cold food may occur.

(1) The Deficient syndromes

① Deficiency of the spleen-yang:

Main manifestations: Sallow and lustreless face, cold feeling over the epigastric region, vomiting of watery fluid, poor appetite, abdominal distension, which is aggravated by eating, desire for hot drinks, loose stool, or emaciation, cold limbs, weak voice and disinclination to talk, pale tongue with whitish coating, soft and weak pulse.

Therapeutic method: Warming and activating yang-qi of the middle-jiao.

Prescription: Lizhong Wan (Bolus for Regulating the Function of the Middle-jiao, from *Treatise on Febrile Diseases*) or the other formulas of this kind.

For cases with cold limbs, Gui Zhi (Ramulus Cinnamomi), Fu Zi (Radix Aconiti), Rou Gui (Cortex Cinnamomi), etc. may be added; for cases with loose stool or frequent defecation with the stool containing the indigested food, Chi Shi Zhi (Halloysitum Rubrum) 15g and Yu Yu Liang (Limonitum) 15g should be added.

② Consumption and deficiency of the spleen-qi (insufficiency of qi of the middle-jiao):

Main manifestations: Anorexia, shortness of breath, disinclination to talk, lassitude of the limbs, borborygmus, abdominal distension, loose stool, or even lowering-down sensation over the lower abdomen, prolapse of the rectum, pale tongue with thin and whitish coating, soft or soft thready pulse.

Therapeutic method: Tonifying the middle-jiao and supplementing qi.

Prescription: Buzhong Yiqi Tang (Decoction for Reinforcing the

Middle-Jiao and Replenishing Qi, from *Treatise on the Spleen and Stomach*) or Renshen Jianpi Wan (Spleen-strengthening Pill of Ginseng, from *A Handbook of Chinese Pharmaceutical Preparation*).

(2) The excessive syndromes

① Cold-dampness disturbing the spleen:

Main manifestations: Epigastric fullness, poor appetite, sticky mouth, heaviness of the head and the body, loose stool, or diarrhea, whitish and greasy coating, soft and thready pulse.

Therapeutic method: Strengthening the spleen to remove dampness or warming up the middle-jiao to remove dampness.

Prescription: Weiling Tang (Stomach Decoction with Poria) or Shipi San (Powder for Reinforcing th Spleen), etc.

Drugs with the action of strengthening the spleen to remove dampness can all be selected in accordance with the patients' conditions.

② Accumulation of dampness-heat in the interior:

Main manifestations: Hypochondiac distension, epigastric fullness, or accompanied with fever, bitter taste in the mouth and thirst, heaviness of the body, dark urine, loose stool, or even yellow coloration of the face and eyes, itching of the skin, yellow and greasy tongue coating, soft and rapid pulse.

Therapeutic method: Clearing away heat and removing dampness.

Prescription: Yinchenhao Tang (Oriental Wormwood Decoction, from *Treatise on Febrile Diseases*), or Yinchen Wuling San (Powder of Wormwood and Five Drugs with Poria, from *Synopsis of Prescriptions of the Golden Chamber*), or the other formulas of this kind.

In addition to the ingredients of the above formula, Hua Shi (Talcum) or Yi Ren (Semen Coicis), etc. can be added to strengthen the spleen and remove dampness; and the drugs relieving the stagnation of the liver -qi such as Yu Jin (Radix Curcumae), Chuan Lian Zi (Fructus Meliae Toosensan) and Qing Pi (Pericarpium Citri Reticulatae Viride) should be adopted together with the above drugs. The proportion of the drugs clearing away heat and those removing damp-

50

ness should be adjusted according to the more dampness or more heat in the treatment of this type.

(3) Combined syndromes

① Deficiency of both the spleen-yang and the kidney-yang:

Main manifestations: Shortness of breath, disinclination to talk, cold limbs, abdominal pain with a cold feeling, or diarrhea at dawn, or borborygmus with watery stool, pale tongue with thin and whitish coating, deep thready pulse.

Therapeutic method: Strengthening the spleen and warming up the kidney.

Prescription: Fuzi Lizhong Tang (Aconite Decoction for Regulating the Middle-jiao, from *Prescriptions of People's Welfare Pharmacy*), Sishen Wan (Pill of Four Miraculous Drugs, from *Standards of Diagnosis and Treatment*), or the other formulas of this kind.

Added by Yi Zhi Ren (Fructus Alpiniae Pxyphyllae), Sishen Wan can be used to treat diarrhea before dawn by taken before sleep. If it is taken long before the diarrhea, the effect will not be satisfactory. In the case of protracted diarrhea due to sinking of qi of the middle-jiao in the debilitated or senile patients, Huang Qi (Radix Astragali seu Hedysari), Dang Shen (Radix Codonopsis Pilosulae), and Bai Zhu (Rhizoma Atractylodis Macrocephalae) should be added to strengthen the spleen and supplement qi.

② The dampness from the spleen attacking the lung:

Main manifestations: Coughing or vomiting sputum or thick fluid, chest fullness, shortness of breath, poor appetite, slightly greasy tongue coating, slippery pulse.

Therapeutic method: Removing dampness and dissolving phlegm.

Prescription: Erchen Tang (Two Old Drugs Decoction, from *Prescriptions of People's Welfare Pharmacy*), Pingwei San (Peptic Powder, from the same book) or the other formulas of this kind.

To the above formulas, Ma Huang (Herba Ephedrae), Xing Ren (Semen Armeniacae Amarum) and Zhi Ke (Fructus Aurantii) can be

51

added to promote dispersion of the lung-qi and dissolve phlegm according to the patients' conditions.

③ Deficiency of both the heart and the spleen: For details, see the Combined syndrome of the heart.

The classifications of the deficiency and excess syndromes of the spleen are relative. In most cases, retention of water and dampness due to dysfunction of the spleen is deficient in origin and excessive in superficials. For the syndrome with more deficiency in origin, the treatment should be aimed at strengthening the spleen, supported by removing dampness, while for that with more dampness, the treatment should be directed at removing dampness, assisted by strengthening the spleen. Moreover, disorders of the spleen are closely related to dampness, whether cold, heat, deficiency or excess syndromes of the spleen can all be accompanied with dampness. Exactly, the cold syndrome of the spleen is often manifested as cold and dampness disturbing the spleen, the heat syndrome as accumulation of dampness-heat in the interior, the excess syndrome as retention of water in the interior, and the deficiency syndrome by hypofunction of the spleen. Therefore, in the selection and application of drugs, the results of syndrome identification and disease diagnosis should be taken into consideration, and drugs for removing dampness, inducing diuresis, eliminating the retained water by loosing the bowel and dissolving dampness should be used deliberately in combination so as to restore the normal function of the spleen by eliminating the dampness. Disorders of the spleen that occur gradually in the development of diabetes, such as the diabetes complicated by diarrhea, diabetic renal disease complicated with edema, and diabetes complicated by hepatitis A, hepatitis B and jaundice, are all closely related to the spleen and dampness. In such cases, in addition to the control of blood sugar and the urine sugar, other accompanying disorders can all be treated with Chinese herbal medicines.

4) Disorders of the stomach

(1) Syndrome of the stomach-cold

Main manifestations: Cold pain over the epigastric region, which is mild but continuous in the mild cases and severe and colic in the severe cases, aggravated by exposure to cold and relieved by warming, tastelessness, no thirst, vomiting watery fluid, hiccup, vomiting, pale tongue with white and moisture coating, deep or slow pulse.

Therapeutic method: Warming the stomach and expelling cold.

Prescription: Liangfu Wan (Galangal and Cyperus Pill) or the formulas of this kind. The selected drugs are Gao Liang Jiang (Rhizoma Alpiniae Officinarum), Xiang Fu (Rhizoma Cyperi), Gan Jiang (Rhizoma Zingiberis, dried), Qing Pi (Pericarpium Citri Reticulatae Viride), Mu Xiang (Radix Aucklandiae), Cao Guo (Fructus Tsaoko), Ding Xiang (Flos Caryophylli, etc.

This is a rare syndrome of diabetes, which may be induced by excessive intake of cool and cold drugs or long-standing use of cold or cool drugs. But vomiting and protracted hiccup are very common in this syndrome, which can be treated by the following drugs: Ding Xiang (Flos Caryophylli) 3g, Shi Di (Calyx Kaki) 3 pieces, Dang Shen (Radix Codonopsis Pilosulae) 12g and Sheng Jiang (Rhizoma Zingiberis Recens) 3 pieces, to be decocted in water for oral use.

(2) Syndrome of the stomach-heat

Main manifestations: Burning pain of the epigastrium, acid regurgitation, gastric discomfort, preference for cold drinks, polyphagia or vomiting right after eating, halitosis, sweeling, pain, ulceration or bleeding of the gums, red tongue with little fluid and yelow coating, slippery rapid pulse.

Therapeutic method: Clearing away heat from the stomach.

Prescription: Qingwei San (Powder for Clearing Away the Stomach-heat, from Secret Record of the Chamber of Orchid) or other formulas of this kind. Drugs to be selected include Huang Lian (Rhizoma Coptidis), Huang Qin (Radix Scutellariae), Sheng Shi Gao (Gypsum Fibrosum), Pu Gong Ying (Herba Taraxaci), Sheng Di

Huang(Radix Rehmanniae), etc.

This is a commonly seen syndrome in diabetics, especially in the early stage of the disease when there are high fever and severe thirst, in a chronic case when bleeding and painful gums due to periodonitis appears. Qingwei San is particularly effective for such cases.

(3) Syndrome of deficiency of the stomach

Main manifestations: Dry mouth and lips, anorexia, or retching and hiccup, dry stool, red tongue with little coating or without coating, thready and rapid pulse.

Therapeutic method: Nourishing the stomach to promote the production of the body fluid.

Prescription: Yiwei Tang(Decoction for Nourishing the Stomach, from *Treatise on Differentiation and Treatment of Epidemic Febrile Diseases*) or the other formulas of this kind. The commonly used drugs include Sha Shen (Radix Adenophorae Strictae), Mai Dong (Radix Ophiopogonis),Sheng Di (Radix Rehmanniae), Yu Zhu(Rhizoma Polygonati Odorati), Shi Hu (Herba Dendrobii), Hua Fen (Radix Trichosanthis),Zhi Mu(Rhizoma Anemarrhenae), etc.

Deficiency of the stomach-yin is very common in diabetics, especially in the senile diabetics. As a result of inadequate intake of water and severe impairment of the yin-fluid, red tongue without coating, etc. may occur, which must be treated with the yin-nourishing drugs so that a better therapeutic effect can be expected.

(4) Syndrome of excess of the stomach

Main manifestations: Epigastric and abdominal fullness and distension, anorexia,beltching or vomiting sour and fetid food,difficult defecation, dirt and greasy tongue coating and slippery pulse.

Therapeutic method: Promoting digestion and removing the stagnated food.

Prescription: Baohe Wan(Lenitive Pill, from *Danxi's Experienmental Therapy*), Zhishi Daozhi Wan(Pill of Immature Bitter Orange for Removing Stagnancy, from *Discussion on the Differentiation of Exogenous*

54

and Endogenous Diseases) or other formulas of this kind. The drugs to be adopted include Shan Zha(Fructus Crataegi), Shen Qu(Massa Fermentata Medicinalis), Mai Ya(Fructus Hordei Germinatus), Gu Ya (Fructus Oryzae Germinatus), Ji Nei Jin (Endothelium Corneum Gigeriae Galli), Zhi Shi (Fructus Aurantii Immaturus),etc.

This syndrome usually arises from improper diet, sudden intake of excessive food, or erroneous intake of contaminiated food. Once it occurs, it should be treated positively, otherwise diabetic ketoacidosis may follow as a result of uncontrolled diet causing aggravation of the disease.

5) Disorders of the liver

(1) Excessive syndromes of the liver

① Stagnation of the liver-qi：

Main manifestations：Hypochondriac pain, hiccup, abdominal pain followed by diarrhea, difficulty in cleaning the anus after defecation, masses,thin tongue coating and wiry pulse.

The hypochondriac pain is marked by a distending and full feeling which may be migratory and lead to inability to turn from one side to another,the hiccup is manifested by frequent belching,and abdominal pain followed by diarrhea and difficulty in cleaning the anus after defecation are due to unrelieved pain in the lower abdomen after defecation, or induced by emotional depression. Mass often appears in the hypochondriac region, on the right or left, or appears and disappears alternately, with stabbing pain occasionally. In addition, this syndrome also displays irritability,poor appetite, etc.

Therapeutic method：Soothing the liver and regulating the circulation of qi, and removing and dissipating masses.

Prescription：Chaihu Shugan San(Buplerum Powder for Relieving Liver-qi,from *Jingyue's Complete Medical Books*), Shixiao San(Wonderful Powder for Relieving Blood Stagnation, from *Prescriptions of People's Welfare Pharmacy*) or other formulas of this kind. The drugs commonly-used are：Chai Hu(Radix Bupleuri), Chuan Lian Zi(Fructus Meliae Toosensan), Xiang Fu (Rhizoma Cyperi), Bai Shao (Radix Paeoniae Alba), Bai Zhu(Rhizoma Atractylodis Macrocephalae), Zhi Ke(Fructus Aurantii), Wu Ling Zhi(Faeces Trogopterorum), Pu Huang(Pollen Typhae), etc. For cases with larger mass, Wa Leng Zi(Concha Arcae), San Leng(Rhizoma Sparagnii),E Zhu (Rhizoma Zedoariae), etc. should be added.

② Flaring-up of the liver-fire:

Main manifestations: Hypochondriac pain, dizziness, headache, sudden and violent rage, tinnitus, deafness, blood-shot eyes, red tongue tip and border, yellow and dry coating, wiry rapid pulse.

Among the symptoms, the dizziness is usually unbearable with throbbing of vessls, the pain occurs in the forehead with hot feeling in this area, and is so severe as if being cut by knife, or with distension. Deafness and tinnitus appear suddenly, paroxymally and cannot be relieved by pressing. In addition, dry stool, dark, hot and difficult urine, flushing of face, bitter taste in the mouth and dry mouth, etc. , may also present.

Therapeutic method: Puring the excessive fire from the liver and the gallbladder.

Prescription: Longdan Xiegan Tang (Decoction of Gentiana for Purging the Liver-fire, from *The Golden Mirror of Medicine*). The drugs to be selected include Long Dan Cao(Radix Gentianae),Zhi Zi (Fructus Gardeniae), Huang Qin (Radix Scutellariae), Mu Tong (Caulis Akebiae), Chai Hu(Radix Bupleuri),etc.

This syndrome is often seen in diabetes with flaring up of the liver-fire, or with dark, scanty and painful urination, pruritus of vulva, eczema of vulva, vulvitis, orchitis, leukorrhagia due to downward flow of dampness-heat from the liver and the gallbladder, or is complicated with urinary infection of excess type, which can all be treated with the above formula. This formula functions to purge the liver-fire and remove dampness and heat. When the liver-fire is purged and the dampness-heat eliminated, the patients' condition will be im-

56

proved and the blood sugar and the urine sugar will be more easily controlled. This formula can not be administered long becaused its effect of purging fire is drastic and the ingredients are bitter in taste and cold in nature which tend to impair the stomach.

③ Up-stirring of the liver-wind:

Main manifestations: Faint, convulsion, numbness, dizziness, wry and tremoring tongue, red tongue tip with thin yellowish coating and wiry rapid pulse. Following the faint, there may be distortion of the eyes and mouth, aphasia and hemiplegia.

Therapeutic method: Suppressing the liver and calming the hyperactive yang, and stopping the wind to relieve convulsion.

Prescription: Tianma Gouteng Yin (Decoction of Gastrodia and Uncaria, from *New Supplement of Diagnosis and Treatment of Miscellaneous Diseases*), or Zhengan Xifeng Tang (Decoction for Tranquilizing the Liver-wind, from *Records of Traditional Chinese and Western Medicine in Combination*).

Formulas of this kind can be adopted for diabetes with hypertension or cerebrovascular diseases.

④ Stagnation of cold in the liver meridian:

Main manifestations: Distending pain in the lower abdomen, distention of scrotum with a lowering-down sensation, or contracture of the scrotum, moist and slippery tongue with whitish coating, deep wiry or deep slow pulse.

Contracture of the scrotum is caused by contraction of the collaterals of the lower abdomen due to accumulation of cold in the liver meridian, therefore, it is usually seen together with distending pain of the lower abdomen. In addition, there may be aversion to cold with the limbs huggled up.

Therapeutic method: Warming up the liver and the liver meridian.

Prescription: Nuangan Jian (Decoction for Warming the Liver Meridian, from Jingyue's Complete Books). As a substitute recipe, equal amount of Xiao Hui Xiang (Fructus Foenicuii), Wu Yao (Radix Linderae) and Chen Xiang (Lignum Aquilariae Resinatum) are to be ground into fine powder to be taken twice after infused in water.

This formula is indicated for excessive cold in the interior marked by pain in the lower abdomen, hernia of cold type, lowering-down sensation of the testis, or cold pain in the lower abdomen in females. It is contraindicated for diabetes manifested as heat syndrome or the syndrome of exuberance of fire due to yin deficiency.

(2) Deficient syndrome of the liver

This is marked by deficiency of the liver and the kidney.

Main manifestations: Dizziness, headache, tinitus, deafness, numbness and tremor of limbs, night blindness, dry red tongue with little fluid and little coating, wiry, thready and rapid pulse.

The tinnitus and deafness occur gradually, the ringing sound is slow and continuous which can be relieved by pressing the ear. In addition, there may be flushed face, red cheeks in the afternoon, insomnia or dream-disturbed sleep.

Therapeutic method: Softening the liver and nourishing the kidney, tonifying yin and suppressing yang.

Prescription: Yiguan Jian (An Ever Effective Decoction, from *Liuzhou's Medical Notes*), Qiju Dihuang Wan (Rehmania Root Decoction with Wolfberry and Chrysanthemum, from *Precious Medical Mirror*), or other formulas of this kind. The drugs commonly used include Gou Qi (Fructus Lycii), Ju Hua (Flos Chrysanthemi), Sheng Di (Radix Rehmanniae), Shan Yao (Rhizoma Dioscoreae), Sha Shen (Radix Adenophorae Strictae), Mai Dong (Radix Ophiopogonis), Dang Gui (Radix Angelicae Sinensis), etc.

This syndrome is very often encountered in diabetics, caused mainly by the consumption of the liver-yin and the kidney-yin in the progression of the diabetes, marked by dry eyes, dizziness and vertigo, eiphora induced by wind. Headache, dizziness or ambiopia caused by hypertension and neurosism can also be treated with Qiju Dihuang Wan, which can also be applied in the form of decoction. Yiguan Jian can be adopted for diabetes complicated with peptic ulcer or chronic hepatitis with pain in the liver region due to fire transformed from stagnated liver-qi following deficiency of the liver-yin and the kidney-yin marked by pain in the chest, hypochondrium and epigastric region, dry throat and tongue, etc.

(3) The combined syndromes

① Disharmony between the liver and the spleen:

Main manifestations: Poor appetite, abdominal distension, borborygmus, loose stool or diarrhea, thin tongue coating, wiry soft pulse.

Therapeutic method: Harmonizing the liver and the spleen.

Prescription: Xiaoyao San (Ease Powder, from *Prescription of People's Welfare Pharmacy*) or the formulas of this kind. The drugs selected to relieve the stagnation of the liver-qi and nourish the liver include Chai Hu (Radix Bupleuri), Bai Shao (Radix Paeoniae Alba), Zhi Ke (Fructus Aurantii) and Dang Gui (Radix Angelicae Sinensis); those used to regulate the function of the spleen are Fu Ling (Poria), Bai Zhu (Rhizoma Atractylodis Macrocephalae), Fo Shou (Fructus Citri Sarcodactylis), Xiang Yuan Pi (Pericarpium Citri), Yi Yi Ren (Semen Coicis), etc.

This syndrome is mainly seen in female diabetics at the climacterium, or the patients with gastrointestinal dysfuction, or those with stagnation of the liver-qi and spleen deficiency due to anger.

② The hyperactive liver-qi attacking the stomach:

Main manifestations: Distension, fullness and pain over the chest and epigastric region, wandering pain of the bilateral hypochondrium, indigestion, eructation, acid regurgitation, thin yellowish tongue coating, wiry pulse.

Therapeutic method: Purging the liver to harmonize the stomach.

Prescription: Chai Hu Shugan San (Liver Qi Dispersing Powder with Radix Bupleuri, from Jingyue's Complete Medical Books) and

Zuojin Wan(Liver Purging Bolus from *Danxi's Experiential Therapy*) in combination or the formulas of this kind. Shugan Hewei Wan(Liver-Dispersing and Stomach-Regulating Bolus) may also be adopted as alternative.

Diabetics with the above symptoms or those with stagnation of the liver-qi due to emotional depression with original spleen deficiency marked by dull pain in the epigastric region can be treated with combined Chaishao Liujunzi Tang (Bupleurum and Peony Decoction of Six Ingredients) and Jinlingzi San(Chinaberry Powder, from *Peaceful Holy Benevolent Prescriptions*).

③ Restlessness of the liver and the gallbladder:

Main manifestations: Restlessness, insomnia, or nightmare with terror and fright, susceptibility to be frightened, shortness of breath, lassitude, blurred vision, bitter taste in the mouth, thin and whitish tongue coating,and deep and thready pulse.

Therapeutic method: Nourishing the liver,clearing away heat from the gallbladder and tranquilizing the mind.

Prescription: Suanzaoren Tang(Wild Jujube Seed Decoction, from *Synopsis of Precsriptions of the Golden Chamber*) or the formulas of this kind. The selected drugs include: Suan Zao Ren (Fructus Ziziphi Spinosae), Huang Lian (Rhizoma Coptidis), Huang Qin (Radix Scutellariae), Bai Shao(Radix Paeoniae Alba),Dang Gui (Radix Angelicae Sinensis), Zhi Zi(Fructus Gardeniae), Chai Hu (Radix Bupleuri),etc.

Diabetics at the early stage or those with latent diabetes marked by frequent irritability and nightmare can be treated with this formula.

④ Deficiency of both the liver-yin and the kidney-yin:

Main manifestations: Wan and withered complexion, flushed cheeks, dizziness, vertigo,dry eyes,soreness and weakness of loins and knees,dry and sore throat, night sweat,feverish sensation over the palms,soles and chest, or difficulty in defecation, emission in males, irregular menstruation or leukorrhagia in females, red tongue without coating, thready rapid pulse.

Therapeutic method: Nourishing yin to purge fire.

Prescription: Dabuyin Wan (Major Bolus for Nourishing Yin, from *Danxi's Experimental Therapy*), or Zhibai Dihuang Wan (Rehmannia Root Bolus with Arnemarrhena and Phellodendron, from *The Golden Mirror of Medicine*), or the other formulas of this kind. Drugs to be adopted are: Zhi Mu (Rhizoma Anemarrhenae), Huang Bai (Cortex Phellodendri), Gou Qi (Fructus Lycii), Ju Hua (Flos Chrysanthemi), Shan Yao (Rhizoma Dioscoreae), Shan Yu Rou (Fructus Corni), Gui Ban (Plastrum Testudinis), Shu Di (Radix Rehmanniae Praeparata), Bie Jia (Carapax Trionycis), etc.

In the case of dry eyes, blurred vision, dizziness and double diplopia, Qiju Dihuang Wan should be adopted. For diabetics with retinal lesions, Mingmu Dihuang Wan (Rehmannia Root Bolus for Improving Eyesight, from *Precious Book of Ophathalmology*) or Shihu Yeguang Wan (Bolus of Dendrobii for Poor Vision, from *Revealing the Mystery of the Origin of Diseases*), both of which function to nourish and tonify the liver and the kidney, and can be applied.

(4) Summary

In brief, the following essential points should be mastered for the treatment of the liver disorders in diabetes:

① The liver is a solid organ, corresponding to wood in the five elements and spring in the seasons. Therefore, the liver-qi tends to go upward and outward, and disorders of the liver are chiefly marked by hyperactivity of the liver-yang. Stagnation and accumulation of cold in the liver meridian is the main cold syndrome of the liver.

② Among the excess syndromes of the liver, depression of the liver-qi, flaring up of the liver-fire and stirring of the liver-wind come from the same source. In other words, they are all related to emotional disturbance.

③ The deficiency syndromes of the liver result mostly from the deficient kidney-yin failing to produce blood and leading to deficiency of the liver-yin and the ensuing hyperactivity of the liver-yang. As the pathogenesis has a close relationship with the deficiency of the kidney-yin, both the liver and the kidney should be treated clinically.

④ The commonly-used therapeutic methods for liver disorders include soothing the liver, clearing away heat from the liver, purging the liver-fire, calming the liver, suppressing the liver, nourishing the liver, softening the liver, warming the liver, etc.

⑤ In recent years, many cases with diabetes have been successfully treated by treating the liver or with the method of relieving the liver depression. Many patients may experience relief of the symptoms of diabetes after being treated with nourishing yin, clearing away heat, supplementing qi or tonifying the kidney, but they still have the syndrome of stagnation of the liver-qi, which is marked by restlessness, insomnia, shortness of breath, dizziness or heaviness of the head, liability to lie flat, lazziness, blurred vision, dry eyes, distension of the hypochondrium, edema of the whole body, or unexpressible discomfort. For these cases, soothing the liver and relieving depression of the liver -qi often result in ease of mind, harmony between qi and blood, and the restoration of health.

6) Disorders of the gallbladder

(1) Excess syndromes of the gallbladder

Main manifestations: Vertigo, deafness, stuffiness of the chest and hypochondriac pain, belching with vomiting of bitter fluid, irritability, restlessness, palpitation, yellow and greasy tongue coating, wiry and slippery pulse.

Therapeutic method: Dissolving the phlegm-heat, regulating the function of the stomach to lower down the adverse flow of the stomach-qi.

Prescription: Huanglian Wendan Tang (Coptis Decoction for Warming the Gallbladder), or other formulas of this kind. The drugs to be adopted are Huang Lian(Rhizoma Coptidis), Huang Qin(Radix Scutellariae), Zhu Ru (Caulis Bambusae in Taeniam), Zhi Shi(Fructus Aurantii Immaturus), Chen Pi(Pericarpium Citri Reticulatae), Ban Xia (Rhizoma Pinelliae), Hou Pu (Cortex Magnolia Officinalis),Yi Yi Ren(Semen Coicis),etc.

No matter what type of diabetes it is, as long as it presents the above symptoms with yellow and greasy coating which indicates dampness-heat in the liver and the gallbladder, the above formula can be employed. When the greasy tongue coating disappears, other formulas may be used, which often decrease the blood sugar and the urine sugar.

(2) The deficiency syndromes of the gallbladder

This is the same with restlessness of the liver and gallbladder.

7) Disorders of the kidney

(1) Deficiency of the kidney-yang

① Unconsolidation of the kidney-qi:

Main manifestations: Pale complexion, soreness and weakness of the lumbus and back, decline of hearing, frequent urination with profuse and clear urine, or even incontinence of urine,or dripping after urine,pale tongue with thin and whitish coating,thready and weak pulse.

Therapeutic method: Strengthening the consolidating effect of the kidney-qi.

Prescription: Dabuyuan Jian(Tonic Decoction for Debility, from *Jingyue's Complete Medical Books*), Mijing Wan(Pill for Reserving the Kidney-essence), etc.

The selected drugs are those tonifying the kidney such as Di Huang (Radix Rehmanniae), Shan Yao(Rhizoma Dioscoreae),Shan Yu Rou(Fructus Corni), Gou Qi(Fructus Lycii), Ren Shen(Radix Ginseng) and Du Zhong (Cortex Eucommiae), and those consolidating the essence such as Duan Mu Li(calcinated Concha Ostreae), Tu Si Zi(Semen Cuscutae), Long Gu(Os Draconis Fossilia), Wu Wei Zi (Fructus Schandrae), Jiu Zi(Semen Allii Tuberosi), and Sang Piao Xiao(Ootheca Mantidis).

63

These formulas are particularly helpful for the senile diabetics who usually have deficiency of the kidey-qi.

② Failure of the kidney to receive qi:

Main manifestations: Shortness and dyspnea aggravated on exertion, perspiration while coughing, incontinence of urine induced by coughing, pale and puffy face, dark tongue with thin and whitish coating, weak pulse.

Therapeutic method: Invigorating the kidney-qi to receive qi.

Prescription: Renshen Hutao Tang(Decoction of Ginseng and Walnut Kernal, from *Prescriptions for Succouring the Sick*), or Shenge San (Powder of Ginseng and Gecko, from *Prescriptions for Universal Relief*).

In the case with asthma due to kidney deficiency or prolonged cough, or hiccup, Qiwei Duqi Wan (All Converging Pill of Seven Drugs) can be applied with modification in order to nourish the kidney and restore the ability of the kidney to receive qi.

③ Insufficiency of the kidney-yang:

Main manifestations: Palish face, soreness and weakness of the loins and knees, impotence, dizziness, tinnitus, aversion to cold, frequent urination, pale tongue with whitish coating, deep weak pulse.

Therapeutic method: Warming up and tonifying the kidney-yang.

Prescription: Yougui Wan (Kidney- Yang- Reinforcing Bolus), Jinkui Shenqi Wan (Bolus of Golden Chamber for Reinforcing the Kidney-qi), or other formulas of this kind. To those formulas, Hai Gou Shen (Panient Testes Callorhini), Ge Jie (Gecko), Dong Chong Xia Cao (Cordyceps), Ba Ji Tian (Radix Morindae Officinalis) and Xian Ling Pi (Herba Epidemii) may be added. For cases with impotence, Xian Ling Pi (Herba Epidemii) and Yang Qi Shi (Actinolitum) should be added; for cases with cold feeling of the waist, Rou Gui (Cortex Cinnamomi) is to be added; and for cases with dripping and profuse urine, Sheng Bai Guo (Semen Ginkgo) and Bu Gu Zhi (Fructus Psoralae) should be supplemented.

④ Overflow of water due to kidney deficiency:

Main manifestations: General edema due to overflow of water to the skin and muscles, which is more severe in the lower legs, distension and fullness of the waist and abdomen, oliguria, or cough with profuse clear sputum and dyspnea due to phlegm formed by the water, pale tongue with whitish coating, deep slippery pulse.

Therapeutic method: Warming up yang to transform water.

Prescription: Zhenwu Tang (Deoction for Controlling Water, from *Treatise on Febrile Diseases*), Jisheng Shenqi Wan (Life Preserving Pill for Replenishing the Kidney-qi, from *Prescriptions for Succouring the Sick*), or other formulas of this kind. The drugs to be selected are: Fu Ling Pi (Cortex Poria), Bai Zhu (Rhizoma Atractylodis Macrocephalae), Bai Shao (Radix Paeoniae Alba), Fu Zi (Radix Aconiti), Ze Xie (Rhizoma Alismatis), Gan Jiang (Rhizoma Zingiberis, dried), Rou Gui (Cortex Cinnamomi), etc.

The above symptoms are usually seen in the later stage of diabetes in which diabetic edema or diabetic renal diseases often occur as a result of deficiency of the spleen-yang and the kidney-yang, and the subsequent overflow of water. In such cases, Jisheng Shenqi Wan or the formulas with similar functions should be administered.

(2) Deficiency of the kidney-yin

① Consumption of the kidney-yin:

Main manifestations: Emaciation, dizziness, tinnitus, insomnia, amnesia, soreness and weakness of the loins and knees, or emission, dry mouth, red tongue with little coating, and thready rapid pulse.

Therapeutic method: Nourishing the kidney-yin.

Prescription: Liuwei Dihuang Wan (Decoction of Six Drugs Including Rehmannia Root), Zuogui Yin (Drink for Tonifying the Kidney-yin), or other formulas of this kind.

② Exuberance of fire due to yin-deficiency:

Main manifestations: Red cheeks and lips, hectic fever, night sweat, soreness of the back and waist, restlessness with insomnia, nocturnal emission, dry mouth and throat, or non-productive cough, dark urine, constipation, red tongue with little coating, thready rapid pulse.

Therapeutic method: Nourishing yin to purge fire.

Prescription: Zhibai Dihuang Wan (Rehmannia Root Decoction with Anemarrhena and Phellodendron) or other formulas of this kind with modifications. The drugs to be selected include Zhi Mu (Rhizoma Anemarrhenae), Huang Bai (Cortex Phellodendri), Di Huang (Radix Rehmanniae), Tian Dong (Radix Asparagi), Mai Dong (Radix Ophiopogonis), Gui Ban (Plastrum Testudinis), etc.

(3) Combined syndromes

① Kidney deficiency and hypofunction of the spleen:

Main manifestations: Loose stool with indigested food, or even incontinence of defecation, abdominal distension, poor appetite, listlessness, aversion to cold, weakness of limbs, pale tongue with thin coating, deep slow pulse.

Therapeutic method: Supplementing the fire (Kidney-yang) to generate earth (the spleen).

Prescription: Fuzi Lizhong Wan (Bolus for Regulating the Middle-jiao with Aconite), Sishen Wan (Pill of Four Miraculous Drugs) or the formulas of this kind. To the formulas, Chi Shi Zhi (Halloysitum Rubrum), Yu Yu Liang (Limonitum), Ke Zi Rou (Fructus Chebulae), Rou Dou Kou (Semen Myristica) may be added; for cases with loose stool, Bai Zhi (Rhizoma Atractylodis Macrocephalae) and Yi Yi Ren (Semen Coicis), etc. should be added.

② Kidney-water attacking the Heart:

Main manifestations: Palpitation, edema, fullness and distension of the chest and abdomen, cough, shortness of breath, inability to lie flat, purplish nails and lips, dark tongue with thin and whitish coating, weak rapid or knotted and intermittent pulse.

Therapeutic method: Warming up the kidney-qi to transform water.

66

Prescription: Zhenwu Tang (Decoction for Controlling Water), Linggui Zhugan Tang (Decoction of Poria, Cinnamon, Bighead Atractylodes and Licorice, from *Treatise on Febrile Diseases*) or the formulas of this kind. Drugs for selection are Gui Zhi (Ramulus Cinnamomi), Fu Ling (Poria), Bai Zhu (Rhizoma Atractylodis Macrocephalae), Ze Xie (Rhizoma Alismatis), Fu Zi (Radix Aconiti), Shao Yao (Radix Paeoniae), Dan Shen (Radix Salviae Miltiorrhizae), etc.

Diabetics with heart failure, edema and inability to lie flat due to dyspnea can be treated with the above formulas.

In the treatment of the kidney disorders, the principle "kidney deficiency should be supplemented but its excess cannot be purged" must be noticed, because it is believed that excess syndromes and exterior syndromes never happen to the kidney. The heat syndrome of the kidney arises from yin deficiency and the cold syndrome of the kidney comes from yang deficiency. For deficiency of the kidney-yin, pungent and dry drugs as well as the drugs bitter in taste and cold in nature should be avoided, instead, it should be treated with the drugs sweet in taste and moisture in nature with the action of tonifying the kidney, so that the sufficient yin will reduce the hyperactive fire and induce the fire to come down. This is what is called "strengthening the water to restrict the hyperactive fire". Yang deficiency is contraindicated for the drugs cool, moisture, pungent and dispersive, it should be treated with those sweet in taste and warm in nature with the action of supplementing qi, so that the sufficient yang can coordinate with yin and eliminate the relatively hyperactive cold. This is what is said: "replenishing yang to expel accumulation of yin". For cases with deficiency of both yin and yang and impairment of both essence and qi, the treatment should be aimed at replenishing both yin and yang.

The lower type of diabetes, senile diabetes or protracted diabetes have a close relationship with disorders of the kidney. Therefore, they can be diagnosed and treated in accordance with the above mentioned and their different manifestations.

3. 3. 3 Types and corresponding treatments of diabetes commonly adopted clinically in modern times

Diabetes is a chronic and progressive disease with unknown causes and multiple complications as well as an extremely slow course, often existing through one's whole life. It is still not so complete and cannot meet the needs of clinical practice to conduct the diagnosis and treatment only in the light of the three types and the theory of zang-fu organs. With the deepening of the research on the causes and pathogenesis of diabetes and the development in its treatment with TCM, new methods of types classification and therapies have arisen one after another. To suit the development and improve the therapeutic effect, the following types often adopted for diagnosis and treatment of diabetes are summarized based on the reports of many doctors in China and the results of long observations and treatment of the disease in Shandong Traditional ChineseMedicine Hospital.

1) Dryness-heat impairing yin(the type marked by exuberant heat in the lung and stomach impairing the yin-fluid)

Main manifestations: Polydipsia, dry mouth and tongue, frequent urination with massive urine or the urine with a sweet taste, polyphagia, emaciation, constipation, red tongue with yellow or dry coating, full rapid or slippery, solid and forceful pulse.

Accompanying symptoms: Erosion of the mouth and tongue, swellon and painful gums, aversion to heat, irritability, halitosis, and bitter taste in the mouth.

Analysis: The lung is an organ with a purifying and descending function and dominates distribution of water. Thus, dryness-heat impairing the lung and consuming the body fluid cause dry mouth and tongue, and polydipsia; direct downward flow of water to the lower-jiao due to failure of the lung-qi to distribute water properly and the ensuing loss of control of the bladder give rise to frequent urination with massive urine or the urine with a sweet taste. The stomach functions to receive and ripen food. Excessive dryness-heat in the stomach will increase the digesting action of the stomach, causing polyphagia and emaciation as a result of the excessive heat consuming and impairing both body fluid and blood. The deficiency of the body fluid in the stomach may cause inability of the large intestine to be moistened, and dryness-heat will accumulate in the large intestine as a result, so there is constipation. In the chronic case, the kidney-yin deficiency and hyperactivity of the kidney-yang due to the further development of the impairment of yin-fluid lead to loss of control of the bladder, so frequent urination with profuse urine occurs and gradually gets worsened. Exuberance of heat in the lung and the stomach is also responsible for red tongue with yellow or dry coating, and full rapid or wiry, solid and forceful pulse.

Therapeutic method: Clearing away heat and promoting the production of the body fluid, and replenishing yin to increase the body fluid.

Prescription: Xiaoke Fang (Formula for Treating Diabetes, from *Danxi's Experiential Therapy*) and Yunu Jian (Gypsum Decoction, from *Jingyue's Complete Medical Books*) in combination with modifications, the ingredients of which are:

Tian Hua Fen (Radix Trichosanthis) 30g, Huang Lian (Rhizoma Coptidis) 10 g, Sheng Shi Gao (Gypsum Fibrosum) 30g, Zhi Mu (Rhizoma Anemarrhenae) 12g, Sheng Di (Radix Rehmannaie) 15g, Mai Dong (Radix Ophiopogonis) 15g, Ge Gen (Radix Puerariae) 20g, Xuan Shen (Radix Scrophulariae) 15g, Niu Xi (Radix Achyranthis Bidentatae) 15g, Sha Shen (Radix Adenophorae Strictae) 15g, and Gan Cao (Radix Glycyrrhizae) 6g.

In Xiaoke Fang, Tian Hua Fen is used in large dose to clear away heat, promote the production of body fluid and quench thirst; Huang Lian, as the assistant, to clear away heat and purge fire; and Sheng Di, Ou Zhi (Liquidom Nelumbinis) and milk to nourish yin, increase fluid and moisten dryness. In Yunu Jian, Shi Gao must be used in large dose to clear away heat from the lung and the stomach, and remove the dryness-heat with its pungent and sweet taste and powerful cold nature; Zhi Mu, bitter in taste and moisture, and cold in nature, to purge both the lung-heat and the stomach-heat and moisten the dryness; Shi Gao, in combination with Zhi Mu can powerfully clear away heat and relieve restlessness; Sheng Di and Mai Dong are used to nourish the stomach-yin and the lung-yin; and Niu Xi to induce the heat to flow downward. Besides, Ge Gen is added to clear away heat, promote the ascending of fluid and treat diabetes so that the effect of promoting the production of body fluid and quenching thirst can be strengthened; Sha Shen and Gan Cao to nourish yin and clear away heat, supplement qi and promote the production of the body fluid. So the above two formulas used in combination can clear away heat, nourish yin, promote the production of the body fluid and increase the body fluid. Clinically, the formulas should be modified flexibly.

Modifications in accordance with symptoms and signs:

① For cases with deficiency of qi and yin of both the lung and the kidney, marked by full, rapid but forceless pulse, severe thirst, frequent urination, and red tongue with little fluid and dry coating, Erdong Tang (Decoctiion of Luciid Asparagus Root and Ophiopogon Root, from *Medicine Comprehended*) should be adopted with modifications. Ingredients of the formula are:

Ren Shen (Radix Ginseng) 6g, Tian Men Dong (Radix Asparagi) 10g, Mai Men Dong (Radix Ophiopogonis) 12g, Tian Hua Fen (Radix Trichosanthis) 30g, Huang Qin (Radix Scutellariae) 6g, Zhi Mu (Rhioma Anemarrhenae) 10g, Gan Cao (Radix Glycyrrhizae) 6g, He Ye (Folium Nelumbinis) 10g, to be decocted in water for oral use.

In this formula, Ren Shen, which may be replaced by Sha Shen (Radix Adenophorae Strictae), functions to supplement qi and promote the production of body fluid; Tian Men Dong, Mai Dong and

Tian Hua Fen to promote the production of body fluid and quench thirst; and Zhi Mu and Huang Qin to clear away heat and purge fire.

② In the Case of severe thirst, preference for cold water, sweating on the head or the upper part of the body, full rapid pulse, dry and yellow tongue coating, which indicate consumption of body fluid and exuberance of heat in the lung and the stomach, the treatment should be directed at clearing away heat from the lung and the stomach, promoting the production of body fluid and supplementing qi with Baihu Jia Renshen Tang (White Tiger Decoction with Ginseng, from *Treatise on Febrile Diseases*), the ingredients of which are:

Sheng Shi Gao (Gypsum Fibrosum) 100g, Zhi Mu (Rhizoma Anemarrhenae) 12g, Gan Cao (Radix Glycyrrhizae Praeparata) 10g, Geng Mi (Polished Glutinous Rice) 12g, Ren Shen (Radix Ginseng) 10g or Sha Shen (Radix Adenophorae Strictae) 20g, to be decocted in water and taken four times or six times.

In this formula, Sheng Shi Gao and Zhi Mu function to clear away heat from the lung and the stomach; and Gan Cao, Geng Mi and Ren Shen to supplement qi, protect the stomach, promote the production of body fluid and quench thirst. These drugs used in combination can remove heat so that the body fluid can be restored. Considering that the exuberant heat in the lung and stomach impairs qi and yin, Ren Shen, which has the function of supplementing qi and nourishing yin, is adopted.

③ In the case of no defecation for several days which indicates accumulation of dryness-heat in the interior and consumption of yin-fluid, the treatment should be aimed to nourish the yin-fluid and moisten dryness to relax the bowel with Zengye Chengqi Tang (Purgative Decoction for Increasing Fluid and Sustaining Qi, from *Treatise on Differentiation and Treatment of Epidemic Febrile Diseases*), which is composed of:

Xuan Shen (Radix Scrophulariae) 30g, Mai Dong (Radix Ophiopogonis) 15g, Sheng Di(Radix Rehmanniae) 15g, Da Huang(Radix seu Rhizoma Rhei) 9g, Mang Xiao(Natrii Sulfas, to be taken after infused in water) 3g, to be decocted in water for oral dose.

④ In the case of exuberance of the stomach-heat, marked by mouth ulcer, swellon and painful gums, bitter taste in the mouth and halitosis, Qingwei San (Powder for Clearing Away the Stomach-heat, from *Secret Records of the Chamber of the Orchids*) should be adopted. The ingredients of the formula are:

Dang Gui(Radix Angeliae Sinensis) 12g, Sheng Di Huang (Radix Rehmanniae) 15g, Mu Dan Pi(Cortex Moutan Radicis) 10g, Sheng Ma(Rhizoma Cimicifugae) 9g, Huang Lian(Rhizoma Coptidis). The drugs added to the formula include Jin Yin Hua (Flos Forsythiae) 30g, Pu Gong Ying(Herba Taraxaci) 30g, and Huang Qin (Radix Scutellariae) 10g.

The above drugs are to be decocted in water for oral dose.

⑤ For cases with diabetic ketosis, Huang Lian(Rhizoma Coptidis) 10g, Huang Qin(Radix Scutellariae) 10g and Sheng Shi Gao(Gypsum Fibrosum) 60g should be added to the formula above, or Xiaotong Tang (Decoction for Reducing Ketone, a proved formula) should be adopted, which consists of:

Huang Qin(Radix Scutellariae) 12g, Huang Lian(Rhizoma Coptidis) 12g, Huang Bai(Cortex Phellodendri) 12g, Zhi Zi (Fructus Gardeniae) 10g, Sheng Di (Radix Rehmanniae) 30g, Dang Gui (Radix Angelicae Sinensis) 20g, Chuan Xiong (Rhizoma Ligustici Chuanxiong) 15g, Fu Ling (Poria) 20g, Pu Gong Ying (Herba Taraxaci) 30g, Sheng Shi Gao(Gypsum Fibrosum) 30g, to be decocted in water for oral dose.

In the case of ketoacidosis, combined Chinese and Western treatment should be administered.

⑥ For cases with pruritus of vulva or itching of the skin, the above formula is to be added with Ku Shen(Radix Sophorae Flavescentis) 12g, Bai Xian Pi(Cortex Dictamni) 12g, and Huang Bai

(Cortex Phellodendri) 9g, and the blood sugar and the urine sugar should be controlled actively.

⑦ In the case of skin infection marked by frequent occurrence of sores and boils, which indicates toxic heat accumulating in the blood, the above formula should be added with Huang Qin(Radix Scutellariae) 12g, Huang Lian(Rhizoma Coptidis) 12g, Pu Gong Ying(Herba Taraxaci) 30g, Ma Chi Xian(Herba Portulacae) 30g and Gan Cao (Radix Glycyrrhizae) 6g. If the skin infection is marked by carbuncles, Wuwei Xiaodu Yin(Antiphlogistic Decoction of Five Drugs, from *The Golden Mirror of Medicine*) can be applied, which consists of:

Jin Yin Hua (Flos Lonicerae) 30g, Ye Ju Hua (Flos Chrysanthemi) 10g, Pu Gong Ying(Herba Taraxaci) 30g, Zi Hua Di Ding(Herba Violae) 12g, Zi Bei Tian Kui Zi(Radix Semiaquilegiae) 12g, to be decocted in water for oral use and the dreg applied to the affected part after being pounded into paste.

At the early stage, diabetes still has a short course. If it is marked by polydipsia, polyphagia and polyuria, especially the former two, which indicate dryness-heat impairing yin, formulas of this kind can be adopted. In most cases, thirst will be markedly relieved after 6 — 15 doses are administered. However, it must be stressed that some of the drugs in these formulas are extremely cold in nature and bitte in taste, so they can not be used long to avoid the dryness transformed from the cold and bitter impairing yin. At this stage, for those who tend to experience hypoglecemia marked by perspiration, hunger, weakness of the body and hands but of their blood sugar and urine glucose or do not have the evident hyperlycemia, they can be treated in accordance with the above method if they are not suitable for or don't want the Western medicines. Some cases of insipidus can also be treated in the same way. Most of the patients will experience remarkable improvement of the symptoms and no side effects will occur. In the selection of formulas and the modifications of the formulas, the drugs clearing away heat, removing toxic materials, activating blood flow and removing blood stasis should be properly added, especially for the treatment in the period after infection or in the presence of blood stasis, in order to raise the therapeutic effects. If the manifestations of deficiency of both qi and yin and blood stasis are evident without obvious dryness-heat in a chronic case, they can be treated in accordance with the treatment for syndrome of deficiency of both qi and yin accompanied with blood stasis.

2) Deficiency of both qi and yin accompanied with blood stasis

Main manifestations: Listlessness, lassitude, lustreless face, shortness of breath, disinclination to talk, spontaneous sweating, or dry throat and tongue, feverish sensation over the palms, soles and chest, or night sweat, flushed face, red tongue with little fluid or with teeth marks or ecchymosis, thready rapid and forceless pulse.

Analysis: Listlessness, lassitude, shortness of breath and disinclination to talk arise from insufficiency of the genuine qi and decline of the functions of the zang-fu organs due to prolonged disease, aging and debility. Failure of the deficient spleen to generate essence and fill the blood into vessels leads to lustreless face. Insufficiency of the lung-qi and the ensuing unconsolidation of the superficies cause shortness of breath and spontaneous sweating. Consumption of the stomach-yin and the lung-yin and the subsequent failure of the yin-fluid to go upward are responsible for dry throat and tongue. Feverish sensation over the palms, soles and chest is due to the internal heat caused by yin-deficiency. The flushed face is ascribed to flaring up of fire due to yin-deficiency, and night sweat is due to the deficient heat forcing the body fluid to be discharged outward. Red tongue with little fluid or with teeth marks, and thready rapid but forceless pulse indicate deficiency of both qi and yin, and obstruction of blood in the collaterals.

Therapeutic method: Supplementing qi and nourishing yin, assisted by activating the blood flow and removing blood stasis.

Prescription: Shengmai San (Pulse-activating Powder, from *Discussion on the Differentiation of Exogenous and Endogenous Diseases*) and Yuye Tang (Decoction for Promoting Production of Body Fluid, from *Records of Traditional Chinese and Western Medicine in Combination*) in combination, which consists of:

Ren Shen (Radix Ginseng) 12g, Mai Dong (Radix Ophiopogonis) 15g, Wu Wei Zi (Fructus Schisandrae) 9g, Sheng Huang Qi (Radix Astragali seu Hedysari) 30g, Ge Gen (Radix Puerariae) 15g, Shan Yao (Rhizoma Dioscoreae) 12g, Ji Nei Jin (Endothelium Corneum Gigeriae Galli) 9g, Zhi Mu (Rhizoma Anemarrhenae) 10g, Hua Fen (Radix Trichosanthis) 30g, Dan Shen (Radix Saliaee Miltiorrhizae) 30g, and Hong Hua (Flos Carthami) 10g, to be decocted in water for oral dose.

In the formula of Shengmai San, Ren Shen, Wu Wei Zi and Mai Dong function to supplement qi, arrest sweating, nourish yin and promote the production of body fluid, so they are indicated for deficiency of both qi and yin marked by profuse sweating, lassitude, shortness of breath, spontaneous sweating, dry mouth and tongue, and thirst, while in Yuye Tang, Huang Qi is used to tonify qi, Ren Shen to tonify the genuine qi, Ge Gen to lift the genuine qi, help to supplement qi and consolidate the superficies to arrest sweating, Shan Yao, Zhi Mu and Hua Fen, used as assistants, to nourish yin and promote the production of body fluid and help yang to rise, and Ji Nei Jin to promote digestion by assisting the spleen. Wu Wei Zi, a common drug of the two formulas, functions to consolidate the kidney-qi and arrest sweating, so that the water will not be distributed downward and outward too much. The above drugs work together to supplement qi, nourish yin, and promote the production of body fluid to quench thirst to restore both qi and yin. Dan Shen and Hong Hua function to activate blood flow and remove blood stasis in this recipe.

Modifications in accordance with the symptoms:

① For cases marked by more qi-deficiency, the above formulas should be used together with Huangqi Yin (Astragalus Root Decoction) in which the dose of Huang Qi (Radix Astragali seu Hedysari)should be as large as 30-60g. In addition, Xi Yang Shen (Radix Panacis Quinquefolii) 12g may be added.

② For cases marked by yin-deficiency, drugs nourishing yin to clear away heat, such as Sheng Di (Radix Rehmanniae) 12g, Shi Hu (Herba Dendrobii) 15g, Sha Shen(Radix Adenophorae) 15g, or Yu Zhu (Rhizoma Polygonati Odorati) 12g, can be added deliberately.

③ For cases with coronary heart disease marked by blood stasis and with ECG changes, Guanxin Erhao (Prescription No. II for CHD) can be adopted.

④ In the case of palpitation, restlessness and insomnia, Chao Zao Ren (Fructus ZIziphi Spinosae, stir-fried) 30g and Bai Zi Ren (Semen Biotae, stir-fried) 15g are to be added to calm the heart and tranquilize the mind.

⑤ For cases with deficiency of both the spleen-qi and the kidney - qi, marked by shortness of breath, disinclination to talk, soreness and weakness of the loins and knees, loose stool, pale tongue with thin whitish coating and deep thready pulse, Shuilu Erxian Dan(Pill of Two Immortals, from *The Collection of Hong's Proved Prescriptions*) and Qianshi Heji (Euryal Seed Mixture) can be adopted jointly, which consist of the following drugs:

Qian Shi(Semen Euryales) 15g, Bai Zhu (Rhizoam Atractylodis Macrocephale) 12g, Shan Yao(Rhizoma Dioscoreae) 12g, Huang Jing(Rhizoma Polygonati) 15g, Tu Si Zi(Semen Cuscutae) 15g, Jin Ying Zi(Rosae Laevigatae) 15g, Bai He (Bulbus Lilii) 15g and Pi Pa Ye(Folium Eriyobotryae) 15g.

Buzhong Yiqi Tang(Decoction for Reinforcing the Middle-jiao and Replenishing Qi, from *Treatise on the Spleen and the Stomach*)can be used with modifications as an alternative, which is composed of:

Ren Shen(Radix Ginseng) 12g, Huang Qi(Radix Astragali seu

Hedysari) 30g, Bai Zhu(Rhizoma Atractylodis Macrocephalae) 15g, Dang Gui(Radix Angelicae Sinensis) 12g, Chen Pi(Pericarpium Citri Reticulatae) 9g, Sheng Ma(Rhizoma Cimicifugae) 9g, Chai Hu (Radix Bupleuri) 9g, Gan Cao(Radix Glycyrrhizae) 6g, Jin Ying Zi(Rosae Laevigatae) 15g, Bu Gu Zhi(Fructus Psoraleae) 15g, and Tu Si Zi(Semen Cuscutae) 20g, to be decocted in water for oral dose.

⑥ For cases with hypertension or dizziness marked by headache, dizziness, tinnitus, insomnia with dream-disturbed sleep, the selected formula is Tianma Gouteng Yin(Drink of Gastrodia and Uncaria, from *Supplement of Diagnosis and Treatment of Miscellaneous Diseses*), which includes:

Tian Ma(Rhizoma Gastrodiae, to be decocted first) 15g, Gou Teng (Ramulus Uncariae cum Uncis, to be decocted later) 18g, Sheng Shi Jue Ming (Concha Haliotidis) 30g, Zhi Zi(Fructus Gardeniae) 10g, Huang Qin (Radix Scutellariae) 10g, Chuan Niu Xi (Radix Achyranthis Bidentatae) 20g, Du Zhong (Cortex Eucommiae) 10g, Yi Mu Cao(Herba Leonuri) 15g, Sang Ji Sheng (Ramulus Loranthi) 15g, Ye Jiao Teng(Caulis Polygoni Multiflori) 20g, Fu Shen(Poria cum Ligno Hospite) 15g, to be decocted in water for oral use.

This formula functions to calm the liver, arrest convulsion, nourish yin and clear away heat, used mainly for headache, dizziness, tinnitus and insomnia caused by hyperactivity of the liver-yang and hypertension. Experiments prove that it can lower the blood pressure.

⑦ In the case of deficiency of the liver-yin and the kidney-yin and hyperactivity of the liver-yang, marked by wan and withered face, dizziness, vertigo, dry eyes, blurred vision, soreness and weakness of the loins and knees, dry and sore throat, emission in males, or irregular menstruation and leukorrahgia in females, red tongue without coating, and wiry thready pulse, the formula to be adopted is

Da Buyin Wan (Major Bolus for Tonifying Yin, from *Danxi's Experiential Therapy*) together with Qiju Dihuang Wan(Rehmannia Root Decoction with Wolfberry and Chrysamthmum, from *Grades of Medicine*) with modifications, and the drugs to be applied are:

Huang Bai(Cortex Phellodendri) 9g, Zhi Mu(Rhizoma Anemarrhenae) 9g, Sheng Di Huang(Radix Rehmanniae) 12g, Gui Ban (Plastrum Testudinis) 30g, Gou Qi Zi(Fructus Lycii) 12g, Ju Hua (Flos Chrysanthemi) 9g, Shan Yu Rou (Fructus Corni) 12g, Shan Yao(Rhizoma Dioscoreae) 12g, Fu Ling(Poria) 15g, Ze Xie(Rhizoma Alismatis) 15g, Dan Pi(Cortex Moutan Radicis) 9g, Shi Hu (Herba Dendrobii) 12g and Hua Fen(Radix Trichosanthis) 30g, to be decocted in water for oral use.

⑧ In the case of yin-deficiency and flaring up of fire marked by nocturnal emission and night sweating, Zhibai Dihuang Wan (Rehmannia Root Bolus with Anemarrhena and Phellodendron, from *Golden Mirror of Medicine*) can be adopted in combination to nourish yin and reduce fire.

⑨ For cases with pulmonary tuberculosis or cough due to yin-deficiency, the original formula can be replaced by Baihe Gujin Tang (Lily Decoction for Strengthening the Lung, from *Collection of Prescriptions with Notes*), which consists of the following drugs:

Shu Di (Radix Rehmanniae Praeparata) 12g, Sheng Di (Radix Rehmanniae)10g, Bei Mu(Bulbus Fritillariae) 10g, Bai He(Bulbus Lilii) 15g, Dang Gui (Radix Angelicae Sinensis) 12g, Chao Shao Yao(Radix Paeoniae, stir-fried) 12g, Xuan Shen(Radix Scrophulariae) 9g, Jie Geng(Radix Platycodi) 9g, Mai Men Dong(Radix Ophiopogonis) 9g, and Gan Cao(Radix Glycyrrhizae) 6g, to be decocted in water for oral use.

This formula functions to nourish yin to clear away heat, moisten the lung and dissolve phlegm.

⑩ For cases with consumption of the heart-qi due to overstrain and exuberance of heart-fire involving the lung, marked by polydipsia and polyuria accompanied with palpitation, dysphoria, tidal fever and thready rapid pulse, the selected formula should be Maimendong Yinzi(Drink of Ophiopogon, from A *Comprehensive Treatise On Prescriptions*) with the following drugs adopted:

Mai Men Dong(Radix Ophiopogonis) 12g, Gua Lou(Fructus Trichosanthis) 24g, Zhi Mu(Rhizoma Anemarrhenae) 12g, Zhi Gan Cao(Radix Glycyrrhizae Praeparata) 6g, Sheng Di Huang(Radix Rehmanniae) 15g, Ren Shen (Radix Ginseng) 9g, Ge Gen(Radix Puerariae) 15g, Fu Shen (Poria cum Ligno Hospite) 15g, Dan Zhu Ye(Herba Lophathemi) 9g, to be decocted in water for oral use.

This formula is indicated for upper type of diabetes marked by polydipsia, chest fullness, dysphoria and shortness of breath.

Deficiency of both qi and yin is the most common pathogenesis of type II diabetes that develops in the adults, which may be manifested as many different patterns or give rise to many complications. In the treatment, Chinese herbal medicine should be taken as the main therapy, supported by the small dose of oral antihyperglycemic such as glybenzcyclamide, etc. , and the formula should be modified in accordance with the blood sugar contents and the changes of the symptoms. In the application of Chinese herbal medicines, the formulas must be properly modified according to the patients' conditions and drugs with the action of activating blood flow and removing blood stasis must be included in any of the formulas applied. The treatment of the accompanying symptoms and complications will be introduced in detail in a special chapter of the book. "Modification in accordance with the symptoms" of this type only refers to the proper modifications of the original formula.

3) Consumption of both yin and yang, and blood stasis in the interior

(1) Main manifestations

① Yin deficiency as the dominant aspect: Dry throat and tongue, feverish sensation over the palms, soles and chest, night sweating.

Because yin deficiency here mainly refers to deficiency of the kidney-yin, there are still dry mouth and sore throat, red cheeks, dizziness, tinnitus, or even deafness, dried and withered helix, wan and withered face, flaccidity of the feet, soreness and weakness of the loins and knees, nocturnal emission in male, irregular menstruation or amenorrhea in female, red tongue with little fluid, deep and thready pulse.

② Yang-deficiency as the dominant aspect: Aversion to cold, cold limbs, soreness and pain of the back and waist, pale complexion, edema of the face and feet, frequent urination with massive urine as turbid as chyme, or urinating twice as much as drinking, or incontinence of urine, nocturnal emission and impotence in male, diarrhea with indigested food, or diarrhea before dawn, dark and enlarged tongue with teeth marks or acchymosis, whitish and moist tongue coating, deep, slow and weak pulse.

Accompanying symptoms: Symptoms of qi-deficiency or deficiency of both qi and yin still exist in this type, and deficiency of both yin and yang may be present, following the qi-deficiency or prolonged yin deficiency which may affect yang.

Analysis: Dry throat and tongue, and sore throat are caused by kidney-yin, deficiency, unremoval of the dryness-heat, and failure of the deficient yin-fluid to go up to moisten the mouth and throat; flaring up of fire due to yin-deficiency leads to red cheeks, deafness, nocturnal emission and amenorrhea; interior heat produced by yin deficiency is responsible for the feverish sensation over the palms, soles and chest; heat due to yin-deficiency forcing the fluid to go outward excessively causes night sweating; lose of nourishment of the muscles and skin due to consumption of the yin-fluid leads to wan and withered face and more frequently the dried and withered helix as the kidney opens into the ears; deficiency of the kidney-yin and insufficiency of the essence and blood failing to supply the lucid orifices on the head lead to dizziness, vertigo and tinnitus; the waist is the house of the kidney, loss of nourishment of the waist due to kidney deficiency causes the soreness and weakness of the loins and the knees, and flaccidity of the feet. Red tongue with little fluid and deep thready pulse all indicate deficiency of the kidney-yin.

Deficiency of the kidney-yang and loss of warmth of the body lead to aversion to cold and cold limbs; the Du Meridian travels through the spinal column, connects with the kidney and controls all yang of the body, so there are cold limbs and soreness, and pain of the back and waist; pale face is due to yang-deficiency and consumption of the kidney-essence; unconsolidation of the kidney-qi due to yang-deficiency leads to emission and impotence which is also a result of relaxation of the tendons in the external genitalia secondary to deficiency of the kidney-yang and decline of the mingmen-fire; uncontrollable urinary orifice due to unconsolidation of the kidney-qi and the ensuing direct downward flow of water bring about frequent urine or incontinence of urine as turbid as chyme with a sweet taste or ketone smell; failure of qi to perform its transforming effect causes sudden discharge of urine in the day time or at night; diarrhea with indigested food and diarrhea before dawn result from inability of the food to be digested due to the declined mingmen-fire unable to generate the earth(spleen) . As a result of the deficiency of the kidney-yang and blood stasis, whitish and moisten tongue coating, deep, slow and weak pulse are present.

Therapeutic method: Nourishing the kidney-yin for that with yin-deficiency as the main aspect; warming up the kidney-yang for that marked by yang-deficiency, and tonifying both yin and yang, replenishing qi and enrichening blood for that characterized by deficiency of yin, yang, qi and blood.

(2) Prescriptions

① For the cases with more yin-deficiency, select Liuwei Dihuang Tang (Decoction of the Six Drugs Including Rehmannia, from *Key to Therapeutics of Childrens' Diseases*) or Zuogui Wan (Pill for Tonifying the Kidney-yin, from *Jingyue's Complete Medical Books*) with modifications. The drugs adopted are:

Shu Di(Radix Rehmanniae Praeparata) 12g, Shan Yao(Rhizoma Dioscoreae) 15g, Shan Yu Rou(Fructus Corni) 12g, Tu Si Zi(Semen Cuscutae) 30g, Gou Qi Zi(Fructus Lycii) 15g, Chuan Niu Xi (Radix Achyranthis Bidentatae) 15g, Lu Jiao Jiao (Colla Cornu Cervi)15g,Gui Ban Jiao(Colla Plastri Testudinis) 15g, to be decocted in water for oral use. Of these drugs, Shu Di, Gou Qi Zi, Shan Yao,Gui Ban Jiao and Niu Xi function to nourish and tonify the kidney-yin, and Shan Yu Rou, Tu Si Zi and Lu Jiao Jiao to tonify the kidney and supplement essence.

② For the cases with more yang-deficiency,select Shenqi Wan(Bolus for Tonifying the Kidney-qi, from *Synopsis of Prescriptions of the Golden Chamber*) or Yougui Wan(Pill for Tonifying the Kidney-yang, from *Jingyue's Complete Medical Books*) with modifications. The drugs to be employed include:

Shu Di Huang (Radix Rehmanniae Praeparata) 12g, Shan Yao (Rhizoma Dioscoreae) 15g, Shan Yu Rou(Fructus Corni) 12g, Gou Qi Zi(Fructus Lycii)15g, Du Zhong(Cortex Eucommiae) 12g, Tu Si Zi(Semen Cuscutae) 30g, Zhi Fu Zi(Radix Aconiti Praeparata) 9g, Rou Gui(Cortex Cinnamomi) 6g, Dang Gui (Radix Angelicae Sinensis) 12g, Lu Jiao Jiao(Colla Cornu Cervi) 15g, to be decocted in water for oral use.

Of these drugs, Fu Zi, Rou Gui and Lu Jiao Jiao, a drug from animal, function to warm and tonify the kidney-yang and supplement essence and marrow, and Shu Di, Shan Yao, Shan Yu Rou, Tu Si Zi,Gou Qi Zi,Du Zhong and Dang Gui to nourish and tonify the kidney and replenish blood and essence with a wonderful effect of nourishing yin to generate yang.

③ For cases with deficiency of yin and yang,and qi and blood,select Lurong Wan(Pill of Pilose Deer Horn, from *Prescriptions Assigned to the Three Categories of the Pathogenic Factors of Diseases*) with modifications. The drugs adopted are:

Lu Rong(Cornu Cervi Pantotrichum) 10g, Ren Shen(Radix Ginseng) 30g, Huang Qi(Radix Astragali seu Hedysari) 60g, Mai Dong (Radix Ophiopogonis) 30g, Wu Wei Zi(Fructus Schisandrae) 20g, Shu Di(Radix Rehmanniae Praeparata) 40g, Rou Cong Rong(Herba Cistanchis) 30g, Xuan Shen(Radix Scrophulariae) 30g, Di Gu Pi (Cortex Lycii Radicis) 30g, Niu Xi (Radix Achyranthis Bidentatae) 15g, Fu Ling(Poria) 40g, Bu Gu Zhi (Fructus Psoraleae) 30g, Shan Yu Rou(Fructus Corni) 30g, Ji Nei Jin(Endothelium Corneum Gigeriae Galli) 15g, to be ground into fine powder and made into pills with water, to be taken 6g each time, three times daily in the morning, at noon and in the evening respectively.

Of the drugs above, Lu Rong is the best drug to warm and tonify the kidney-yang, Ren Shen and Huang Qi function to tonify the kidney-qi to assist yang-qi, and the other drugs to nourish yin, clear away heat and supplement both qi and blood. This is a patent drug that can be taken long but does not bring about harm to the body. If there is no such patent products, the formula may vary according to the patients' conditions and be made into pills with water for oral use. If it is administered in the form of decoction, Fu Pen Zi(Fructus Rubi), Sang Piao Xiao(Ootheca Manitis) and Jin Ying Zi(Rosae Laevigatae)may be added to tonify the kidney and strengthen the consolidating effect of the kidney.

(3) Modifications in accordance with symptoms

① For cases with heat due to yin-deficiency, marked by severe thirst, add Hua Fen (Radix Trichosanthis) 30g, Huang Lian (Rhizoma Coptidis)10g and Ge Gen(Radix Puerariae)15g, to clear away heat from the upper-jiao, promote the production of body fluid and quench thirst.

② For cases with exuberant fire due to yin-deficiency, marked by tidal fever, dry mouth, sore throat, and red tongue, add Zhi Mu(Rhizoma Anemarrhenae), Huang Bai(Cortex Phellodendri)and Di Gu

Pi(Cortex Lycii Radicis) to nourish yin and reduce fire.

③ For cases with deficiency of the kidney-yin and yin deficiency affecting yang, marked by insomnia, dream-disturbed sleep, dysphoria, irritability, complicated by unconsolidation of the kidney- qi marked by nocturnal emission and premature ejaculation, the treatment should be aimed at tonifying the kidney and supplementing essence, consolidating the kidney-qi and arresting emission. The formula should be added with Long Gu(Os Draconis), Mu Li(Conch Ostreae), Jin Ying Zi(Rosae Laevigatae), Qian Shi(Semen Euryales), Lian Xu(Stamen Nelumbinis), Gui Ban(Plastrum Testudinis), and Bie Jia (Carapax Trionycis), or used together with Jinsuo Gujing Wan(Golden Lock Pill for Keeping the Kidney -essence, from *Collections of Prescriptions with Notes*) or Shuilu Erxian Dan(Pill of Two Immortals, from *Standards of Diagnosis and Treatment*),to promote the consolidating effect of the kidney and arresting emission.

④ For cases with impotence associated with pale, dizziness, vertigo, soreness and weakness of loins and knees, listlessness, inability to erect the penis or to make the penis hard while having intercourse, pale tongue with whitish coating and deep thready pulse, which indicate decline of the kidney-yang and decline of the mingmen fire, Wuzi Yanzong Wan(Pill of Seeds of Five Drugs for Treating Masculine Sterility, from *Danxi's Experiential Therapy*) or Zanyu Dan(Bolus for Reproduction, from *Jingyue's Complete Books*) can be adopted with modifications.

⑤ For cases with edema marked by general edema which is more serious under the waist, tastlessness, loose stool, cold limbs, enlarged tongue with whitish coating, deep thready and forceless pulse, caused by deficiency of both qi and yin of both the spleen and the kidney and the subsequent overflow of water, the treatment should be to supplement qi, strengthen the spleen, tonify the kidney and induce diuresis. For the mild cases with edema and oliguria, the above formula should be added with Fu Ling(Poria),Fu Ling Pi(Cortex Poria),

Fu Ping (Herba Spirodelae) and Che Qian Zi (Semen Plantaginis) to induce diuresis and treat edema; for cases due to yang deficiency and the ensuing overflow of water, Shipi San (Powder for Strengthening the Spleen-yang, from *Revision of Prescriptions for Succouring the Sick*) can be employed with modification.

Edema is a commonly-seen symptom in the patients with advanced diabetes. Generally speaking, this formula can be used at the first step in the treatment of edema of any causes. The diabetes complicated by renal disease will be discussed in a special chapter of this book.

⑥ If this type is marked by blood stasis in pathogenesis, Dan Shen (Radix Salviae Miltiorrhizae), Chi Shao (Radix Paeoniae Rubra), Tao Ren (Semen Persicae), Hong Hua (Flos Carthami) and Chuang Xiong (Rhizoma Ligustici Chuanxiong) should be added to activate blood flow and remove blood stasis.

⑦ Lingering diarrhea, marked by diarrhea with undigested food, or diarrhea before dawn, pale complexion, pale and enlarged tongue proper with teeth prints and deep slow pulse, indicates decline of the mingmen-fire, failure of the earth (spleen) to be generated and the ensuing inability of the spleen to digest food. For the treatment of diarrhea with undigested food, nourishing, oily or lubricating drugs should be reduced from the formula, and Dang Shen (Radix Codonopsis Pilosulae), Bai Zhu (Rhizoma Atractylodis Macrocephalae) and Yi Yi Ren (Semen Coicis) should be added to supplement qi, strengthen the spleen, induce diuresis and stop diarrhea; for the diarrhea before dawn caused by deficiency of both the spleen-yang and the kidney-yang, Sishen Wan (Pill of Four Miraculous Drugs, from *Standards of Diagnosis and Treatment*) may be adopted in combination to warm up the spleen and kidney, astringe the intestine and stop diarrhea.

⑧ For cases with weakness of the kidney-yang and inability of the kidney to receive qi marked by dyspnea and shortness of breath which would be more severe on exertion, Zuogui Wan (Pill for Tonifying

the Kidney-yin) can be adopted with Bu Gu Zhi(Fructus Psoraleae),
Wu Wei Zi (Fructus Schisandrae)and Ge Jie(Gecko)to tonify the
kidney and help the kidney to receive qi.

Yin and yang of the human body are mutually dependent. Yang-
deficiency often develops from the advancement of qi-deficiency or
yin-deficiency and is characterized by the symptoms of interior cold,
which are more serious than those of the qi-deficiency or the yin deficiency. Deficiency of the heart-yang, deficiency of the spleen-yang
and deficiency of the kidney-yang are the most commonly encountered types of yang-deficiency. As the kidney-yang is the basis of
yang-qi of the whole body, deficiency of the heart-yang or the
spleen-yang will eventually involve the kidney-yang,leading to deficiency of both the heart-yang and kidney-yang or deficiency of both
the spleen-yang and the kidney-yang. If deficiency of both yin and
yang develops further, depletion of yin and exhaustion of yang or
even isolation of yin and yang will ensue, and death will occur finally. As the syndrome mostly comes from impairment of yin by dryness-heat, impairment of both qi and yin and yin-deficiency affecting yang, blockage of this development with proper treatment will
make the disease stablised and the patients' lives prolonged.

4) Obstruction of dampness-heat in the middle-jiao

Main manifestations: Dry mouth with preference for large amount
of drinks, abdominal fullness and distension after drinking, or thirst
but not desire for drinking, sweet taste in the mouth with a sticky
feeling, polyphagia, or sometimes eating little with gastric discomfort
and hungry, fat physique, edema in the lower limbs, listlessness,las-
situde, heaviness of the head and body, dark red tongue with thick
and greasy or yellow,thick and greasy coating,soft and rapid pulse.

Analysis: Diseases caused by pathogenic dampness may be either
exogenous or endogenous. Dampness-heat obstructing in the middle-
jiao is mostly caused by affection of exogenous dampness, and improper diet or excessive intake of fat, sweet or alcohol, which pro-

86

duces dampness-heat and the accumulation of the dampness-heat in the spleen and stomach. It may also be caused by long-standing use of cold or cool drugs in the treatment of exuberant dryness-heat at the early stage of the disease, which leads to impairment of the spleen and stomach, failure of the spleen to transform and transport water and dampness, and the ensuing transformation of heat from the stagnated dampness. As a result of dampness disturbing the spleen, the spleen is not able to transform water into the body fluid and send it up, so there are polydipsia, or thirst but not desire for drinks and sweet taste in the mouth with a sticky feeling; the spleen-deficiency and exuberance of dampness cause abdominal distension and fullness, gastric discomfort after eating or hungry; retention of dampness in the interior is responsible for heaviness of the head and the body, fat physique or even edema in the lower limbs; and dark red tongue indicates the complicated blood stasis. Thick and greasy or yellow thick and greasy tongue coating suggest obstruction of dampness-heat in the interior.

This syndrome is neither a commonly-encountered nor an essential syndrome of diabetes. But it may be common in the transmission of the disease or in the diabetes with complications.

Therapeutic method: Clearing away heat and removing dampness.

Prescription: Huangqin Huashi Tang (Scutellaria and Talc Decoction, from *Treatise on Differentiation and Treatment of Epidemic Febrile Diseases*) with modifications. The drugs to be adopted are:

Huang Qin (Radix Scutellariae) 12g, Hua Shi (Talcum) 15g, Fu Ling (Poria) 12g, Da Fu Pi (Pericarpium Arecae) 9g, Bai Kou Ren (Semen Amomi Cardamomi) 10g, Tong Cao (Medulla Tetrapanacis) 3g, Zhu Ling (Polyporus) 15g, Huang Lian (Rhizoma Coptidis) 10g, Hou Pu (Cortex Magnolia Officinalis) 10g, Pei Lan (Herba Eupatorii) 12g, and Shi Chang Pu (Rhizoma Acori Graminei) 12g, to be decocted in water for oral use.

In the formula, Huang Lian and Huang Qin function to clear

away heat and dry the dampness; Fu Ling, Hua Shi and Zhu Ling to remove the dampness by inducing diuresis; Hua Shi also functions to clear away heat and remove dampness; Bai Kou Ren, Da Fu Pi and Hou Pu function to promote the flow of qi, remove dampness and relieve abdominal fullness and distension; Tong Cao to clear away heat and induce diuresis; Shi Chang Pu to remove dampness and regulate the function fo the stomach; and Pei Lan to dissolve the turbid-dampness with its aromatic taste. This formula is indicated for dampness-heat in the middle-jiao and therefore it can be used with proper modification to treat diabetes with dampness-heat in the middle-jiao. With the removal of the dampness-heat, other manifestations of diabetes will also show improvement. In addition to the above formula, diabetes with dampness-heat in the middle-jiao can be also treated with Ermiao San (Two Wonderful Drugs Powder, from *Danxi's Experiential Therapy*), Yueju Wan (Pill for Relieving Stagnancy, from the same book as above), Lianpu Yin (Coptis-Magnolia Drink, from *On Severe Vomiting with Diarrhea*), or Ganlu Xiaodu Dan (Sweet Dew Detoxication Pill, from *Compendium on Epidemic Febrile Diseases*), etc. As dampness-heat in the middle-jiao is a deteriorated case of diabetes, attentions should also be paid to the original diabetes in the treatment, in other words, both the original and secondary conditions of the disease should be treated at the same time.

Modifications in accordance with the symptoms:

① For cases with obstruction of dampness and spleen deficiency, caused by endogenous generation of dampness following spleen-yang deficiency, or by stagnation of cold-dampness in the middle-jiao following deficiency of the spleen-qi and stomach-qi, which is marked by sallow face, lassitude, listlessness, fullness and distension of the epigastrium and abdomen, anorexia, eructation, or aversing to fat and greasy food, loose stool or diarrhea, greasy tongue coating and soft pulse, Xiangsha Liujunzi Tang (Decoction of Cyperus and Amomum with Six Noble Ingredients, from *Collection of Prescriptions with*

Notes) can be employed to strengthen the spleen, remove dampness and regulate the function of the stomach, which can also be used to treat diabetes complicated with chronic gastritis and peptic ulcer with the above symptoms. The drugs to be applied are:

Dang Shen (Radix Codonopsis) 15g, Bai Zhu (Rhizoma Atractylodis Macrocephalae) 12g, Fu Ling (Poria) 12g, Mu Xiang (Radix Aucklandiae) 9g, Sha Ren (Fructus Amomi) 9g, Ban Xia (Rhizoma Pinelliae) 9g, Chen Pi (Pericarpium Citri Reticulatae) 9g, Gan Cao (Radix Glycyrrhizae) 6g, Bai Kou Ren (Semen Amomi Cardamomi) 12g, and Yi Yi Ren (Semen Coicis) 15g, to be decocted in water for oral use.

② For cases of cold-dampness disturbing the spleen, caused by exposure to cold or excessive intake of raw and cold food or drinks leading to stagnation of cold-dampness in the middle-jiao, or by the original exuberance of dampness in the interior disturbing the yang-qi of the middle-jiao and the ensuing generation of cold-dampness in the middle-jiao, and manifested as fullness of the epigastrium and abdomen, poor appetite, nausea, vomiting, tastelessness in the mouth with no thirst, abdominal pain with loose stool, heaviness feeling of the head as being wrapped with a cloth, heaviness or edema of the body, whitish and greasy tongue coating, soft and slow pulse, the treatment should be aimed at warming up the middle-jiao and removing dampness with Weiling Tang (Stomach Decoction with Poria, from *Danxi's Experiential Therapy*) or Shipi San (Powder for Reinforcing the Spleen, from *Revision of Prescriptions for Succouring the Sick*) with modifications. The drugs to be adopted are:

Cang Zhu (Rhizoma Atractylodis) 12g, Hou Pu (Cortex Magnolia Officinalis) 9 g, Chen Pi (Pericarpium Citri Reticulatae) 6g, Bai Zhu (Rhizoma Atractylodis Macrocephalae) 10g, Fu Ling (Poria) 12g, Zhu Ling (Polyporus) 12g, Ze Xie (Rhizoma Alismatis) 10g, Gui Zhi (Ramulus Cinnamomi) 6g, Gan Cao (Radix Glycyrrhizae) 3g, Sheng Jiang (Rhizoma Zingiberis Recens) 3 pieces, and Da Zao

(Fructus Ziziphi Jujubae) 5 pieces, to be decocted in water and taken twice.

This syndrome is not common in the development of diabetes, but it may be seen frequently in the transmission of the disease or in the case with complications, especially in the critical case complicated by cancers. This is a syndrome that is very difficult to treat and by now there is still no radical therapy. So it is helpful to study the ancient's understanding and stress "Diseases may present visible manifestations and deteriorated conditions and may transform into other diseases in the course of their developement. Thus formulas should be administered based on an overall understanding of the developement of the diseases." This is a practical method of analysing the deteriorated cases or the accompanying syndromes and complications of diabetes, and the author adevocate the use of the formulas mentioned above in the treatment of critical diabetes with white and greasy tongue coating which does not respond to Western therapy.

3. 4 The commonly-used therapeutic methods

3. 4. 1 Clearing away heat, moistening the lung and promoting the production of the body fluid to quench thirst

The commonly adopted prescriptions: Tian Hua Fen (Radix Trichosanthis) 30g, Huang Lian (Rhizoma Coptidis) 10g, Sheng Di (Radix Rehmanniae) 12g, Zhi Mu (Rhizoma Anemarrhenae) 10g, Mai Dong (Radix Ophiopogonis) 15g, Ge Gen (Radix Puerariae) 20g, Wu Wei Zi (Fructus Schisandrae) 9g, Tai Zi Shen (Radix Pseudostellariae) 30g, etc. The representative of these formulas is Xiaoke Fang (Prescriptions for Diabetes) combined with Yuquan San (Jade Fountain Powder).

Indication: The upper type of diabetes manifested as polydipsia, dry mouth and tongue, frequent urination with massive urine, red tongue tip and border, thin and yellow tongue coating, full and rapid pulse.

90

3. 4. 2 Purging the stomach-fire, nourishing yin and preserving body fluid

The commonly adopted prescriptions: Sheng Shi Gao (Gypsum Fibrosum) 30 — 60g, Zhi Mu (Rhizoma Anemarrhenae) 12g, Sheng Di (Radix Rehmanniae) 15g, Mai Dong (Radix Ophiopogonis) 15g, Xuan Shen (Radix Scrophulariae) 15g, Huang Lian (Rhizoma Coptidis) 10g, Niu Xi (Radix Achyranthis Bidentatae) 15g. The representative of such formulas is Yunu Jian (Gypsum Decoction).

Indications: The miidle-type of diabetes marked by polyphagia, emaciation, constipation, dry and yellow tongue coating, slippery, solid and forceful pulse.

3. 4. 3 Nourishing yin and consolidating the kidney-qi

The commonly adopted prescriptions: Sheng Di (Radix Rehmanniae) 12g, Shu Di (Radix Rehmanniae Praeparata) 12g, Shan Yao (Rhizoma Dioscoreae) 15g, Shan Yu Rou (Fructus Corni) 12g, Ze Xie (Rhizoma Alismatis) 10g, Dan Pi (Cortex Moutan Radicis) 10g, Fu Ling (Poria) 10g, Tai Zi Shen (Radix Pseudostellariae) 30g, Qian Shi (Semen Eurgales) 15g, Jin Ying Zi (Rosae Laevigalatae) 20g, etc. The representative of such formulas is Liuwei Dihuang Wan (Bolus of Six Drugs Including Rehmannia).

Indication: The lower-type of diabetes due to consumption of the kidney-yin marked by frequent urination with massive urine, or the urine as turbid as chyme or with a sweet taste, dry mouth and tongue, red tongue and deep thready pulse.

3. 4. 4 Warming up the kidney and supplementing yang

The commonly adopted prescriptions: Gou Qi Zi (Fructus Lycii) 15g, Tu Si Zi (Semen Cuscutae) 30g, Wu Wei Zi (Fructus Schisandrae) 9g, Fu Pen Zi (Fructus Rubi) 15g, Che Qian Zi (Semen Plantaginis) 30g, Bu Gu Zhi (Fructus Psoraleae) 12g, Xian Ling Pi (Herba Epimedii) 12g, Ba Ji Tian (Radix Morindae Officinalis) 12g, Xian Mao (Rhizoma Curculiginis) 10g, Yang Qi Shi (Actinolitum) 12g, etc. The representative of such formulas is Wuzi Yangzong

Wan(Pill of Seeds of Five Drugs for Treating Masculine Sterility).

Indications: Diabetes complicated with yang deficiency manifestations such as impotence and premature ejaculation, juvenile senilism or sterility with cold sperms.

3. 4. 5 Warming and nourishing the kidney to induce astringency

The commonly adopted prescriptions: Fu Zi(Radix Aconoti) 9g, Rou Gui (Cortex Cinnamomi) 9g, Shu Di (Radix Rehmanniae Praeparata) 15g, Shan Yao (Rhizoma Dioscoreae) 15g, Shan Yu Rou(Fructus Corni) 15g, Fu Ling(Poria) 12g, Ze Xie(Rhizoma Alismatis) 12g, Sang Piao Xiao(Ootheca Mantidis) 12g, and Wu Wei Zi(Fructus Schisandrae) 9g. The Representative of such formulas is combined Jinkui Shengqi Wan(Bolus of Golden Chamber for Tonifying the Kidney-qi)and Sangpiaoxiao San(Mantis Egg-case Powder).

Indications: The lower-type of diabetes due to deficiency of both the kidney-yin and the kidney-yang, marked by frequent urination turbid as chyme, or even urinating twice as much as drinking, dark and lustreless face, dry and withered helix, soreness and weakness of the loins and knees, or even impotence, pale tongue with whitish coating, deep thready and forceless pulse.

For cases with edema of the face and the lower limbs, add Che Qian Zi (Semen Plantaginis) 30g, Ze Lan(Herba Lycopi) 30g and Fang Ji(Radix Stephaniae Tetrandrae) 12g.

3. 4. 6 Supplementing qi and strengthening the spleen

The commonly adopted prescriptions: Huang Qi(Radix Astragalus seu Hedysari) 30g, Ren Shen(Radix Ginseng) 10g, Ban Xia(Rhizoma Pinelliae) 10g, Zhi Gan Cao(Radix Glycyrrhizae Praeparata) 10g, Qiang Huo(Rhizoma seu Radix Notopterygii) 10g, Du Huo (Radix Angelicae Dahuricae) 12g, Bai Shao(Radix Paeoniae Alba) 10g, Fang Feng(Radix Ledebouriellae) 10g, Chen Pi(Pericarpium Citri Reticulatae) 9g, Fu Ling(Poria) 12g, Bai Zhu (Rhizoma Atractylodis Macrocephalae) 12g, Ze Xie(Rhizoma Alismatis) 12g, Huang Lian (Rhizoma Coptidis) 10g, Sheng Jiang (Rhizoma Zingiberis Recens) 3 pieces, and Da Zao(Fructus Ziziphi Jujubae) 5 pieces. The representative of the formulas is Qiwei Baizhu San(Powder of Seven Drugs with Bighead Atractylodes, from *Key to Therapeutics of Children's Diseases*).

Indications: Deficiency of both the stomach-qi and the spleen-qi due to long-standing hypofunction of the spleen and stomach and consumption of the body fluid, marked by polydipsia, poor appetite, emaciation, lassitude, listlessness, loose stool, pale tongue with thin and whitish coating, deep, thready and forceless pulse.

Clinically, if there are heaviness feeling of the body and limbs, lassitude with desire for lie flat, aversion to wind and cold limbs, bitter taste in mouth, dry tongue, and indigestion, which indicate sinking of qi due to spleen-deficiency, the treatment should be to lift the spleen-yang with Shengyang Yiwei Tang(Decoction for Elevating the Spleen-yang and Nourishing the Stomach, from *Treatise on the Spleen and Stomach*).

3.4.7 Relieving depression of the liver-qi assisted by purging the liver-fire

The commonly-adopted prescriptions: Dan Pi(Cortex Moutan Radicis) 10g, Zhi Zi(Fructus Gardeniae) 10g, Chai Hu(Radix Bupleuri) 10g, Zhi Shi(Fructus Aurantii Immaturus) 10g, Chi Shao(Radix Paeoniae Rubra) 10g, Bai Shao(Radix Paeoniae Alba) 10g, Fu Ling(Poria) 10g, Xuan Shen(Radix Scrophulariae) 15g, Hua Fen (Radix Triochosanthis) 30g, Huang Lian(Rhizoma Coptidis) 10g, Dang Gui(Radix Angelicae Sinensis) 12g, Bo He(Herba Menthae) 9g, and Gan Cao(Radix Glycyrrhizae) 6g. The representative formula: Danzhi Xiaoyao San(Ease Powder of Moutan Bark and Cape Jasmine Fruit, from *Prescriptions of People's Welfare Pharmacy*).

Indications: Dysphoria with tinnitus, dry mouth and thirst, bitter taste in mouth, polydipsia, polyphagia and dry stool.

3.4.8 Activating blood flow and removing blood stasis

The commonly-adopted prescriptions: Huang Qi(Radix Astragali seu Hedysari) 30g, Chi Shao(Radix Paeoniae Rubra) 15g, Chuan Xiong(Rhizoma Ligustici Chuanxiong) 10g, Dang Gui(Radix Angelicae Sinensis) 20g, Di Long (Lumbricus) 10g, Tao Ren(Semen Persicae) 10g, Hong Hua (Flos Carthami) 10g, Dang Shen (Radix Codonopsis Pilosulae) 15g, Mai Dong(Radix Ophiopogonis) 12g, Sheng Di(Radix Rehmanniae) 20g, and Shi Hu(Herba Dendrobii) 12g. The representative formula is Buyang Huanwu Tang(Decoction of Invigorating Yang for Recuperation, from *Corrections on the Errors of Medical Works*).

Indications: Polydipsia accompanied with chest stuffiness, shortness of breath, numbness and pain of limbs, or apoplexy with paralysis, difficulty in limb movement, dark lips, dark tongue with ecchymosis, engorgement of the sublinguinal veins with a purple colour, thready uneven or knotted and intermittent pulse.

For climacteric syndrome in female, the formula to be selected is Erxian Tang (Decoction of Curculigo Rhizome and Epimedium, a proved formulas in the Shanghai Hospital of Shuguang, from *A Handbook of Commonly-Used Formulas*) with modifications. The selected drugs are: Xian Mao Gen(Rhizoma Curculiginis) 12g, Xian Ling Pi (Herba Epimedii) 12g, Ba Ji Tian (Radix Morindae Officinalis) 6g, Huang Bai (Cortex Phellodendri) 9g, Zhi Mu (Rhizoma Anemarrhenae) 9g, and Dang Gui(Radix Angelicae Sinensis) 9g, to be decocted in water for oral dose. This formula is indicated for climacteric syndrome, climacteric hypertension, amenorrhea and other diseases marked by insufficiency of both the kidney-yin and the kidney-yang with flaring up of fire of the deficiency-type. Experiment proved that this formula has a remarkable effect of lowering experimental hypertension.

Chapter 4　Classifications of the Commonly-used Formulas and Herbs

According to records in the medical literature from the ancient to the modern times, the commonly-used Chinese herbs for treating diabetes are classified as follows:

4. 1 The commonly-used Chinese herbs in clinic

4. 1. 1 Classification of Chinese herbs

1) Diaphoretics

Exterior syndrome designates the diseases caused by exogenous pathogens, which is marked by chills and fever. The diaphoretics have the property of dispersion, thus applicable to the exterior syndromes caused by exogenous pathogens. When a diabetic presents chills, fever and other manifestations of an exterior syndrome due to invasion of exogenous pathogens, he or she should be treated with the diaphoretics.

The diaphoretics in TCM include: Zi Su (Fructus Perillae), Jing Jie (Herba Schizonepetae), Bai Zhi (Radix Angelicae Dahuricae), Fang Feng (Radix Ledebouriellae), Sheng Jiang (Rhizoma Zingiberis Recens), Niu Pang Zi (Fructus Arctii), Sang Ye (Folium Mori), Ju Hua (Flos Chrysanthemi), Ge Gen (Radix Puerariae), Sheng Ma (Rhizoma Cimicifugae), Chai Hu (Radix Bupleuri), Fu Ping (Herba Spirodelae), Dou Chi (Semen Sojae Preparatum), etc.

2) Heat-clearing drugs

The drugs that are bitter in taste and cold in nature with the action of clearing away heat are called heat-clearing drugs, which can be subdivided into heat-clearing and fire-purging drugs, heat-clearing and blood-cooling drugs, heat- clearing and dampness- removing drugs, and heat-clearing and detoxicating drugs. These drugs can be used coordinatively in the clinic according to patients' conditions.

The commonly-used heat-clearing drugs include: Zhi Mu (Rhizoma Anemarrhenae), Shi Gao(Gypsum Fibrosum), Tian Hua Fen (Radix Trichosanthis), Lu Gen(Rhizoma Phragmitis), Zhi Zi(Fructus Gardeniae), Dan Zhu Ye(Herba Lophatheri), Huang Lian(Rhizoma Coptidis), Huang Qin(Radix Scutellariae), Sheng Di (Radix Rehmanniae), Xuan Shen(Radix Scrophulariae), Di Gu Pi(Cortex Lycii Radicis),Chi Shao(Radix PAeoniae Rubra),Lian Qiao(Fructus Forsythiae), Ma Chi Xian (Herba Portulacae), Dan Pi (Cortex Moutan Radicis), Yin Chai Hu (Radix Stellariae), Bai Mao Gen (Rhzoma Imperatae), Pu Gong Ying (Herba Taraxaci), Di Ding (Herba Violae),Da Qing Ye(Folium Isatidis).

3) Antirheumatics

Any drug that can be used to treat obstruction of the meridians and the ensuing impeded circulation of qi and blood by eliminating the pathogenic wind-dampness from the meridians, tendons and bones falls into this group. These drugs have the effect of relieving arthralgia caused by wind and dampness.

The commonly-used antirheumatics include: Du Huo(Radix Angelicae Pubscentis), Qin Jiao(Radix Gentianae Macrophyllae), Cang Zhu(Rhizoma Atractylodis), Mu Gua(Fructus Chaenomelis), Wei Ling Xian(Radix Clematidis), Sang Zhi(Ramulus Mori), Sang Ji Sheng(Ramulus Loranthi). Shen Jin Cao(Herba Lycopodii), Cang Er Zi (Fructus Xanthii), and Hu Zhang (Rhizoma Polygoni Cuspidati). In addition to treating rheumatism, some of these drugs such as Cang Zhu and Cang Er Zi, still have the effect of lowering the blood sugar, and the drugs with the action of relaxing muscles and tendons, including Mu Gua, Wei Ling Xian and Shen Jin Cao can aslo be used to treat diabetes complicated by arthralgia manifested as difficulty in movement and heel pain.

4) Cold-expelling drugs

These drugs include Fu Zi(Radix Aconiti), Rou Gui(Cortex Cinnamomi), Gan Jiang(Rhizoma Zingiberis),Wu Zhu Yu(Fructus Euodiae), Xiao Hui Xiang (Fructus Foenicuii) and Bi Bo (Fructus Piperis Longi). They are usually adopted for the diabetes with cold manifestations due to yang deficiency, but are not so frequently used in most cases.

5) Purgatives

Drugs included in this group are: Da Huang(Radix seu Rhizoma Rhei), Mang Xiao(Natrii Salfus),Huo Ma Ren(Fructus Cinnabis), Yu Li Ren(Semen Pruni) and Fan Xie Ye(Folium Cassiae),which can be used as supplements when diabetes presents constipation or difficult defecation in the aged patients.

6) Diuretics

These drugs include Fu Ling(Poria), Zhu Ling(Polyporus), Ze Xie(Rhizoma Alismatis), Chi Xiao Dou(Semen Phaseoli), Yi Yi Ren(Semen Coicis), Yu Mi Xu(Stigma Maydis), Deng Xin Cao (Medulla Junci), Che Qian Zi (Semen Plantaginis), Hua Shi (Talcum),Zhu Ye(Lophatherum),Yin Chen(Herba Artemisiae),Shi Wei(Folium Pyrrosiae),Bi Xie(Rhizoma Dioscoreae Septemlobae) and Dong Gua Pi(Exocarpium Binincasae).

These drugs function to induce diuresis to eliminate dampness, so they are often adopted to treat edema, oliguria or jaundice complicated by urinary diseases.

7) Sedatives

Sedatives in TCM include: Long Gu(Os Draconis), Mu Li(Concha Ostreae), Zhen Zhu Mu(Margarita), Zi Shi Ying(Fluoritum), Bai Zi Ren(Semen Biotae), Yuan Zhi(Fructus Polygalae), He Huan Pi(Cortex Albiziae)and Ye Jiao Teng(Caulis Polygoni Multiflori).

These drugs can be selected to treat pre-pulsation marked by palpitation with nightmare in early diabetes or vegetative nerve functional disturbance to transquilize mind and relieve restlessness.

8) Drugs for Regulating Flow of Qi

This group include Xiang Fu(Rhizoma Cyperi), Mu Xiang(Radix Aucklanidae), Li Zhi He(Semen Litchi), Zhi Ke(Fructus Aurantii), Hou Pu(Cortex Magnolia Officinalis), Sha Ren(Fructus Amomi), Bai Dou Kou (Semen Amomi Cardamomi), Mei Gui Hua (Flos Rosae) and Chai Hu(Radix Bupleuri), which can be selected to treat diabetes complicated by depression of the liver-qi with epigastric fullness and distension.

9) Drugs for Calming the Liver to Stop Wind

These drugs include: Tian Ma(Rhizoma Gastrodiae), Gou Teng (Ramulus Uncariae cum Uncis), Bai Ji Li(Fructus Tribuli), Ci Shi (Magnetitum), Shi Jue Ming(Concha Haliotidis), Di Long(Lumbricus), Jiang Can(Bombyx Batryticatus), Quan Xie(Scorpio), and Wu Gong(Scolopendra).

This group of drugs has the effect of calming the liver, checking hyperactive yang and tranquilizing the wind, often used to treat the diabetic complications of hypertension, dizziness, headache, numbness and pain in limbs, etc.

10) Drugs for Treating Blood Disorders

The diseases of the blood system includes blood-deficiency, blood-heat, blood stasis, and bleeding, which should be treated with the therapeutic methods nothing more than enriching the blood for blood-deficiency, removing heat from the blood for blood-heat, promoting circulation of blood for blood stasis, and arresting bleeding for bleeding. The drugs for enriching the blood and removing heat from the blood belong to tonics and heat- clearing drugs respectively. This group of drugs mainly refer to those for activating blood flow by removing blood stasis and those for arresting bleeding. The commonly-used drugs are: Chuan Xiong(Rhizoma Ligustici Chuanxiong), Dan Shen (Radix Salviae Miltiorrhizae), Tao Ren (Semen Persicae), Hong Hua(Flos Carthami), Yi Mu Cao(Herba Leonuri), Ze Lan (Herba Lycopi), San Leng(Rhizoma Sparganii), E Zhu (Rhizoma Zedoariae), Yu Jin(Radix Curcumae), Jiang Huang(Rhizoma Curcumae Longae), Yuan Hu (Rhizoma Corydalis), Wu Ling Zhi(Faeces Trogopterori), Jiang Xiang(Lignum Dalbergiae Odoriferae), Niu Xi (Radix Achyranthis Bidentatae), Ji Xue Teng (Caulis Spatholobi), Liu Ji Nu(Herba Artemisiae Anomalae), Yue Ji Hua (Flos Rosae Chinensis), Pu Huang(Pollen Typhae), Xian He Cao (Herba Agrimoniae), Bai Ji(Rhizoma Bletillae), San Qi(Radix Notoginseng), Xiao Ji(Herba Cephalanoploris), Qian Cao Gen(Radix Rubiae), etc.

This group of drugs may be selected as supplements to treat any type of diabetes in the treatment with Chinese drugs, especially complications such as coronary heart disease, angina pectoris, retinopathy and renal lesions corresponding to the pathologic change of micrangium, or the tendency to bleeding.

11) Tonics

This group of drugs include: Ren Shen (Radix Ginseng), Dang Shen(Radix Codonopsis Pilosulae), Tai Zi Shen(Radix Pseudostellariae), Huang Qi(Radix Astragali seu Hedysari), Shan Yao(Rhizoma Dioscoreae), Bai Zhu(Rhizoma Atractylodis Macrocephalae),Huang Jing(Rhizoma Polygonati), Bian Dou(Semen Dolichoris), Dang Gui (Radix Angelicae Sinensis), Shu Di (Radix Rehmanniae Praeparata), He Shou Wu(Radix Polygoni Multiflori), Gou Qi Zi (Fructus Lycii), Bai Shao(Radix Paeoniae Alba), Sang Shen(Fructus Mori), Tu Si Zi(Semen Cuscutae), Tian Men Dong(Radix Asparagi), Xuan Shen(Radix Scrophulariae), Mai Dong(Radix Ophiopogonis), Shi Hu(Herba Dendrobii), Yu Zhu(Rhizoma Polygonati Odorati), Lu Rong (Cornu Cervi Pantotrichum), Lu Jiao (Cornu Cervi), Lu Jiao Jiao(Colla Cornus Cervi), Lu Jiao Shuang(Cornu Cervi Degelatinatum), Ba Ji Tian(Radix Morindae Officinalis), Xian Ling Pi (Herba Epimedii), Xian Mao Gen (Rhizoma Curculiginis), Rou Cong Rong(Herba Cistanchis), Yi Zhi Ren(Fructus Alpiniae Oxyphyllae), Bu Gu Zhi(Fructus Psoraleae), Chuan Duan(Radix Dipsaci), Du Zhong(Cortex Eucommiae), Sha Yuan

Zi(Semen Astragali Complanati), Hu Lu Ba(Semen Trigonellae), Han Lian Cao(Herba Ecliptae), and Nu Zhen Zi(Fructus Ligustri Lucidi).

This group of drugs includes the drugs for invigorating qi, enrichening the blood, tonifying yin, and invigorating yang, suitable for the treatment of the deficiency of both qi and blood, and the deficiency of both yin and yang. They are able to strengthen the physiological function of the organism, or to supplement deficiency of the human body. When there appears the deficiency of both qi and blood in diabetes, these drugs are often employed.

12) Astringents

These drugs include: Wu Wei Zi(Fructus Schisandrae), Wu Bei Zi(Galla Chinensis), Wu Mei(Fructus Mume), Shan Zhu Yu(Fructus Corni), Sang Piao Xiao(Ootheca Mantidis), Fu Pen Zi(Fructus Rubi), Ying Su Ke(Involucrum Castaneae), Long Gu(Os Draconis Fossilia), Mu Li(Concha Ostreae), and Jin Ying Zi(Rosae Laevigatae).

When diabetics present unconsolidation of the kidney-qi due to kidney deficiency marked by enuresis, emission, urinary protein, and hyperglycosuria, these drugs can be administered to consolidate the kidney to retard urine.

4.1.2 A survey of the study of some drugs

Ren Shen(Radix Ginseng) has a remarkable inhibiting effect on rabbits' hyperglycemia induced by injection of adrenalin and lupertonic glucose, and a hypoglycemic effect on both normal dogs and the dogs of alloxan diabetes. Its roots, stalks and leaves have an effect on the normal blood sugar of rabbits and rats, but can evidently reduce the hyperglycemia caused by hypertonic glucose injection, and the high dose(100mg/kg) has much clearer effect which remains for 1—2 weeks after stopping using the drug.

Huang Qi(Radix Astragali seu Hedysari) can not only exert a tonic effect on the heart to induce diuresis, reduce blood pressure and sugar, abate angiocardiopathy accompanying diabetes, but also resist bacteria, diminish inflammation, and eliminate various infections caused by metabolic disorder.

Huanglian Shuijian Ji(Coptis Decoction) can reduce the blood sugar of the normal mice. The main effective ingredient, Rhizoma Coptidis-berberine, can reduce the blood sugar of the normal mice, the mice of alloxan diabetes and the KK mice of spontaneous diabetes. Berberine can resist the increase of the blood sugar caused by the injection of glucose, inhibit glyconeogensis taking alanine as substrate, and its effect has a close relation with the increase of blood lactate. Therefore, it may produce the effect of reducing blood sugar through glyconeogenesis and/or the promotion of glucolysis.

Ge Gen(Radix Puerariae) has the effect of reducing blood sugar. Puerarin is the main active ingredient of Radix Puerariae, and administration of puerarin by 50mg /kg can obviously reduce the blood sugar.

Zhi Mu(Rhizoma Anemarrhenae) mainly contains saponin, can reduce blood sugar and the Ketone bodies in urine, and make the death rate less than that in the contrast group through the experiments on animals.

Li Zhi He(Semen Litchi) can effectively reduce the blood sugar index of the rats of alloxan hyperglycemia. The subcutaneous injection of 60—40mg/kg of the extractum of Semen Litchi to the mice can reduce the blood sugar and also the content of hepatic glycogen evidently.

Kugua Zhiji(Momordica Charantia Praeparata) has an evident effect of reducing blood sugar on both the normal animals and the animals of alloxan hyperglycemia, and has a strong power to combine with insulin receptor and insulin antibody. Hypoglycemi mechanism drawn from Kugua Zhiji Praeparata may be that the active mass contains para-imsulin.

Sheng Di(Radix Rehmanniae), Dang Shen(Radix Codonopsis Pilosulae) and the extractum of Sheng Di (Radix Rehmanniae) all have the evident effect of reducing blood sugar when given by subcutaneous injection or by oral dose to the normal rabbits. The blood sugar may clearly rise by the subcutaneous injection of the extractum of Dang Shen (Radix Codonopsis Pilosulae) to the normal rabbits, but it may not rise or may fall a little by the injection of Dang Shen (Radix Codonopsis Pilosulae) together with the extractum of Sheng Di (Radix Rehmanniae).

Through the experimental study of seven pairs of drugs often used in the treatment of diabetes, Tian Hua Fen (Radix Trichosanthis) and Zhi Mu (Rhizoma Anemarrhenae), Cang Zhu (Rhizoma Atractylodis) and Xuan Shen (Radix Scrophulariae), Huang Qi (Radix Astragali seu Hedysari) and Shan Yao (Rhizoma Dioscoreae), Sheng Di (Radix Rehmanniae) and Dan Pi (Cortex Moutan Radicis), and Mai Dong (Radix Ophiopogonis) and Wu Wei Zi (Fructus Schisandrae) all have evident effect on the inhibition of the normal mice's blood sugar, of which the pair of Tian Hua Fen (Radix Trichosanthis) and Zhi Mu (Rhizoma Anemarrhenae) has the fastest, strongest and longest, being the first. Its effect of reducing blood sugar has no obvious difference from that of D860.

Through the pharmacological experiments, Sheng Di (Radix Rehmanniae), Mai Dong (Radix Ophiopogonis), Xuan Shen (Radix Scrophulariae), Shan Yao (Rhizoma Dioscoreae), Fu Ling (Poria) and Cang Zhu (Rhizoma Atractylodis) have the effect of reducing blood sugar, and can inhibit the experimental hypergalycemia; Wu Bei Zi (Galla Chinensis), Sheng Long Gu (Os Draconis) and Sheng Mu Li (Concha Ostreae) can contract the blood vessels of the intestinal walls and inhibit the intestinal walls from absorbing glucose, thus reducing the ingestion of sugar.

4. 2 The commonly-used formulas in clinic

4. 2. 1 The cmmonly-used ancient famous formulas

1) The formulas for invigorating qi and clearing away heat

(1) Renshen Baihu Tang (White Tiger Decoction of Ginseng, from *Prescriptions of Peaceful Benevolent Dispensary*)

Ingredients: Tian Hua Fen (Radix Trichosanthis), Huang Lian (Rhizoma Coptidis), Sheng Di (Radix Rehmanniae), Ou Zhi (Liquidom Nelumbinis Rhizomatis), a moderate amount of milk, Mai Dong (Radix Ophiopogonis), Ge Gen (Radix Puerariae), to be decocted in water for oral dose.

Functions: Clearing away heat to moisten the lung, and promoting the production of body fluid to quench thirst.

(2) Zhuye Shigao Tang (Lophatherum and Gypsum Decoction, from *Treatise on Febrile Diseases*)

Ingredients: Zhu Ye (Lophatherum), Shi Gao (Gypsum Fibrosum), Ban Xia (Rhizoma Pinelliae), Mai Men Dong (Radix Ophiopogonis), Ren Shen (Radix Ginseng), Zhi Gan Cao (Radix Glycyrrhizae Praeparata), and Geng Mi (Semen Oryzae).

Preparation: Stew the first six drugs with one liter of water, get the decoction 600ml, remove the dregs, then cook Geng Mi (Semen Oryzae) with the decoction until the decoction is well done, then remove Geng Mi (Semen Oryzae). Divide it into two shares, to be taken warm twice.

Fuctions: Clearing away heat to promote the production of body fluid, and supplementing qi to regulate the stomach.

(3) Maimendong Yinzi (Ophiopogon Drink, from *A Comprehensive Treatiseon Prescription*)

Ingredients: Mai Men Dong (Radix Ophiopogonis, with the core removed), Gua Lou (Fructus Trichosanthis), Zhi Mu (Rhizoma Anemarrhenae), Gan Cao (Radix Glycyrrhizae Praeparata), Sheng Di (Radix Rehmanniae), Ren Shen (Radix Ginseng), Ge Gen (Radix Puerariae), and Fu Shen (Poria cum Ligno Hospite).

Preparation and administration: Grind the above drugs into fine powder to be taken 15g each time. Or decoct the above in proper amount of water until 150ml of the decoction is got, removed the dregs and take the decoction warm after meal.

Functions: Supplementing qi and promoting the production of body fluid.

(4) Yu Quan Wan(Jade Fountain Pill, from *Renzhai Effective Prescriptions*)

Ingredients: Mai Dong (Radix Ophiopogonis, core removed and dried in the sun), Ren Shen (Radix Ginseng), Fu Ling (Poria), Huang Qi(Radix Astragali seu Hedysari, incompletely processed and honeyed), Wu Mei(Fructus Mume, baked), Gan Cao(Radix Glycyrrhizae), Tian Hua Fen (Radix Trichosanthis), and Ge Gen (Radix Puerariae).

Preparation: Grind the drugs above into fine powder, make bolus of the size of a pellet with honey to be taken one bolus once after chewed with warm water.

Functions: Supplementing qi to nourish yin and promoting the production of body fluid to quench thirst.

(5) Xiaoke Fang(Prescription for Diabetes, from *Danxi's Experiential Therapy*)

Ingredients: Huang Lian Mo(Rhizoma Coptidis, powdered), Tian Hua Fen Mo(Radix Trichosanthis, powdered), Sheng Di Zhi(Succus Rehmanniae), Ou Zhi (Liquidom Nelumbinis Rhizomatis), human milk, Jiang Zhi(Succus Zingiberis), and Mel, to be decocted in water for oral dose.

Functions: Clearing away heat to moisten the lung and promoting the production of body fluid to quench thirst.

(6) Yuye Tang(Decoction for Promoting Production of Body Fluid, from *Records of Traditional Chinese and Western Medicine in Combination*)

Ingredients: Shan Yao(Radix Dioscoreae), Huang Qi(Radix Astragali seu Hedysari), Zhi Mu(Rhizoma Anemarrhenae), Ji Nei Jin (Endothelium Corneum Gigeriae Galli), Ge Gen(Radix Puerariae),

104

Wu Wei Zi (Fructus Schisandrae), and Tian Hua Fen (Radix Trichosanthis), to be decocted in water for oral dose.

Functions: Supplementing qi to nourish yin and promoting the production of body fluid to quench thirst.

2) The formulas for nourishing yin and clearing away heat

(1) Bai Hu Tang (White Tiger Decoction, from *Treatise on Febrile Diseases*)

Ingredients: Shi Gao (Gypsum Fibrosum), Zhi Mu (Rhizoma Anemarrhenae), Zhi Gan Cao (Radix Glycyrrhizae Praeparata), and Geng Mi (Semen Oryzae).

Preparation: Decoct the above drugs in water until Geng Mi is well-done, then remove the dreg. Take the decoction warm.

Function: Clearing away heat and promote the production of body fluid.

(2) Yunu Jian (Gypsum Decoction, from *Jingyue's Complete Medical Books*)

Ingredients: Sheng Shi Gao (Gypsum Fibrosum), Shu Di (Radix Rehmanniae Praeparata), Mai Dong (Radix Ophiopogonis), Zhi Mu (Rhizoma Anemarrhenae), and Niu Xi (Radix Achyranthis Bidentatae).

Preparation: Be decocted in 300ml water to get 200ml of the decoction and orally taken either warm or cool.

Functions: Removing heat from the stomach and nourishing yin.

(3) Yiguan Jian (An Ever Effective Decoction for Nourishing the Liver and Kidney, from *Liuzhou's Medical Notes*)

Ingredients: Bei Sha Shen (Radix Glehniae), Mai Dong (Radix Ophiopogonis), Dang Gui (Radix Angelicae Sinensis), Sheng Di (Radix Rehmanniae), Gou Qi Zi (Fructus Lycii), and Chuan Lian Zi (Fructus Meliae Toosendan).

Preparation: Decoct the drugs above in water, remove the dregs and take the decoction orally while it is warm.

Functions: Nourishing yin and regulating the liver-qi.

(4) Zuogui Yin (Drink for Tonifying the Kidney-yin, from *Jingyue's Complete Medical Books*)

Ingredients: Shu Di (Radix Rehmanniae Praeparata), Shan Yao (Rhizoma Dioscoreae), Gou Qi Zi (Fructus Lycii), Zhi Gan Cao (Radix Glycyrrhizae Praeparata), Fu Ling (Poria), and Shan Yu Rou (Fructus Corni), to be decocted in water for oral dose.

Functions: Tonifying yin and the kidney.

3) The formulas for tonifying the kidney and arresting polyuria

(1) Shenqi Wan (Bolus for Tonifying the Kidney-qi, from *Synopsis of Prescriptions of the Golden Chamber*)

Ingredients: Sheng Di (Radix Rehmanniae), Shan Yao (Rhizoma Dioscoreae), Shan Yu Rou (Fructus Corni), Ze Xie (Rhizoma Alismatis), Fu Ling (Poria), Mu Dan Pi (Cortex Moutan Radicis), Gui Zhi (Ramulus Cinnamormi), and Fu Zi (Radix Aconiti Praeparata).

Preparation: Mix the drugs together, grind them into fine powder, make boluses with honey each of which weighs 15g, to be taken with boiled water in the morning and evening, one bolus each time.

Functions: Warming and tonifying the kidney-yang.

(2) Yougui Yin (The Kidney-Yang-Reinforcing Decoction, from *Jingyue's Complete Medical Books*)

Ingredients: Shu Di (Radix Rehmanniae Praeparata), Shan Yao (Rhizoma Dioscoreae), Shan Yu Rou (Fructus Corni), Gou Qi Zi (Fructus Lycii), Gan Cao (Radix glycyrrhizae Praeparata), Du zhong (Cortex Eucommiae), Rou Gui (Cortex Cinnamomi), and Zhi Fu Zi (Radix Aconiti Praeparata).

Preparation: To be decocted in water for oral dose.

Functions: Warming the kidney and replenishing essence.

(3) Suoquan Wan (Pill for Reducing Urination, from *The Effective Prescriptions for Women*)

Ingredients: Wu Yao (Radix Linderae) and Yi Zhi Ren (Fructus Alpiniae Oxyphyllae).

Administration: Take 6g of the pills each time with boiled water,

106

one or twice a day.

Functions: Warming the kidney, dispelling cold, and arresting polyuria and enuresis.

4) The formulas for promoting blood circulation by removing blood stasis

(1) Xuefu Zhuyu Tang(Decoction for Removing Blood Stasis in the Chest, from *Corrections on the Errors of Medical Works*)

Ingredients: Tao Ren (Semen Persicae), Hong Hua (Flos Carthami), Dang Gui(Radix Angelicae Sinensis), Sheng Di(Radix Rehmanniae), Chuan Xiong(Rhizoma Ligustici Chuanxiong), Chi Shao(Radix Paeoniae Rubra), Niu Xi (Radix Achyranthis Bidentatae), Jie Geng(Radix Platycodi), Chai Hu(Radix Bupleuri), Zhi Ke(Fructus Aurantii), and Gan Cao(Radix Glycyrrhizae).

Preparation: Decoct the above drugs in water for oral dose.

Functions: Promoting blood circulation by removing blood stasis and promoting circulation of qi to relieve pain.

(2) Tao Hong Siwu Tang (Decoction of Four ingredients with Peach Kernel and Safflower, from *The Golden Mirror of Medicine*)

Ingredients: Shu Di (Radix Rehmanniae Praeparata), Chuan Xiong (Rhizoma Ligustici Chuanxiong), Chi Shao (Radix Paeoniae Alba), Dang Gui(Radix Angelicae Sinensis), Tao Ren(Semen Persicae), and Hong Hua(Flos Carthami).

Preparation: Decoct the above drugs in water to be taken at three times within a day.

Functions: Nourishing blood, promoting blood circulation and removing blood stasis.

4.2.2 The commonly-used formulas in the modern reports

(1) Huoxue Jiangtang Fang(The Formula for Promoting Blood Circulation and Reducing Blood Sugar, from *Journal of Beijing Traditional Chinese Medicine College*; 1986,(5): 27)

Ingredients: Huang Qi(Radix Astragali seu Hedysari), Shan Yao (Rhizoma Dioscoreae), Cang Zhu (Rhizoma Atractylodis), Xuan

Shen (Radix Scrophulariae), Dang Gui (Radix Angelicae Sinensis), Chi Shao (Radix Paeoniae Rubra), Chuan Xiong (Rhizoma Ligustici Chuanxiong), Yi Mu Cao (Herba Leonuri), Dan Shen (Radix Salviae Miltiorrhizae), Ge Gen (Radix Puerariae), Sheng Di (Radix Rehmanniae), Shu Di (Radix Rehmanniae Praeparata), and Mu Xiang (Radix Aucklandiae).

Preparation: To be decocted in water for oral dose.

Functions: Supplementing qi, nourishing yin, promoting blood circulation, and removing obstruction in the channels.

(2) Danggui Huoxue Tang (Chinese Angelica Decoction for Promoting Blood Circulation, from *New Traditional Chinese Medicine*; 1985; (4): 29)

Ingredients: Dang Gui (Radix Angelicae Sinensis), Dan Shen (Radix Salviae Miltiorrhizae), Chi Shao (Radix Paeoniae Rubra), Hong Hua (Flos Carthami), Xuan Shen (Radix Scrophulariae), and Ren Dong Teng (Caulis Lonicerae).

Preparation: To be decocted in water for oral dose.

Functions: Promoting blood circulation, and clearing away heat and toxic materials.

(3) Zishen Rongjing Wan (Pill for Nourishing the Kidney-essence, from *Hunan Journal of Traditional Chinese Medicine*; 1987, (6): 8)

Ingredients: Huang Jing (Rhizoma Polygonati), Rou Cong Rong (Herba Cistanchis), Zhi Shou Wu (Radix Polygoni Multiflori Praeprata), Jin Ying Zi (Rosae Laevigatae), Huai Shan Yao (Rhizoma Dioscoreae Huaishanyao), Chi Shao (Radix Paeoniae Rubra), Shan Zha (Fructus Crataegi), Wu Wei Zi (Fructus Schisandrae), and Tablet of Finger Citron.

Preparation: Bake and dry the drugs above, grind them into powder, make boluses with water, coat the boluses with the Charcoal ash of the haw powder, and polish and dry them. Take the boluses 6g each time, three times daily, and 30 days for one course of treatment.

Functions: Nourishing the kidney, consolidating the origin, invigorating the liver and kidney, promoting blood circulation, and removing obstruction in the channels.

(4) Shenggan Tang (Decoction for Lowering Blood Sugar, from *Shandong Journal of Traditional Chinese Medicine*; 1988, (2):27)

Ingredients: Shan Yu Rou (Fructus Corni), Wu Wei Zi (Fructus Schisandrae), Wu Mei (Fructus Mume), and Cang Zhu (Rhizoma Atractylodis).

Preparation: Decoct the herbs above in water 2000ml to get 1000ml of decoction, to be taken warm before meals, three times daily.

Functions: Inducing astringency, nourishing yin and removing dryness.

(5) Buyin Guse Tang (Decoction for Tonifying Yin and Inducing Astringency, from *The Traditional Chinese Medicine of Guangxi*; 1989, (3):18)

Ingredients: Sheng Di (Radix Rehmanniae), Xuan Shen (Radix Scrophulariae), Mu Dan Pi (Cortex Moutan Radicis), Lian Xu (Stamen Nelumbinis), Tian Hua Fen (Radix Trichosanthis), Huang Qi (Radix Astragali seu Hedysari), Long Gu (Os Draconis Fossilia Ossis Mastodi), Mu Li (Concha Ostreae), Gou Qi Zi (Fructus Lycii), Shan Yu Rou (Fructus Corni), and Wu Wei Zi (Fructus Schisandrae).

Preparation: To be decocted in water for oral dose.

Functions: Tonifying yin and inducing astringency.

(6) Tangniao Bing Yihao Heji (Mixture No. 1 for Diabtetes, from *The Journal of Traditional Chinese Medicine*; 1989, (7))

Ingredients: Sheng Di (Radix Rehmanniae), Shu Di (Radix Rehmanniae Praeparata), Huang Lian (Rhizoma Coptidis), Tian Dong (Radix Asparagi) Mai Dong (Radix Ophiopogonis), Xuan Shen (Radix Scrophulariae), Da Fu Pi (Pericarpium Arecae), Fu Ling

(Poria), Zhi Mu (Rhizoma Anemarrhenae), Wu Wei Zi (Fructus Schisandrae), Shan Yu Rou (Fructus Corni), Dang Shen (Radix Codonopsis Pilosulae,) Huang Qi (Radix Astragali seu Hedysari), and Shi Gao (Gypsum Fibrosum).

Preparation: Make concentracted mixture (1g in each ml) with the medicines above, 500ml a bottle. The mixture is taken orally, 50—80ml each time, three times daily, half an hour before meals, and 3 months for one course of treatment.

Functions: Nourishing yin, clearing away heat, tonifying the kidney, and inducing astringency.

(7) Tangniaobing Fang (Prescription for Diabetes, from *The Journal of New Medicine and Pharmacy*; 1976, (5))

Ingredients: Huang Qi (Radix Astragali seu Hedysari), Shan Yao (Rhizoma Dioscoreae), Cang Zhu (Rhizoma Atractylodis), Xuan Shen (Radix Scrophulariae), Sheng Di (Radix Rehmanniae), Mai Dong (Radix Ophiopogonis), Dang Shen (Radix Codonopsis Pilosulae), Wu Wei Zi (Fructus Schisandrae), Fu Ling (Poria), Wu Bei Zi (Galla Chinensis), Mu Li (Concha Ostreae), and Long Gu (Os Draconis Fossilia Ossis Mastodi).

Preparation: To be decocted in water and taken one dose three times a day.

Functions: Nourishing yin, clearing away heat, and invigorating the spleen and qi.

(8) Yitang Tang (Decoction for Controlling Diabetes, from *Jilin Traditional Chinese Medicine*; 1983, (5):22)

Ingredients: Shi Gao (Gypsum Fibrosum), Shan Yao (Rhizoma Dioscoreae), Mai Dong (Radix Ophiopogonis), Tian Hua Fen (Radix Trichosanthis), Shu Di (Radix Rehmanniae Praeparata), Shi Hu (Herba Dendrobii), Bi Xie (Rhizoma Dioscoreae Septemlobae), Qian Shi (Semen Euryales), Fu Pen Zi (Fructus Rubi), Tu Si Zi (Semen Cuscutae), Sang Piao Xiao (Ootheca Mantidis), Yi Zhi Ren (Fructus Alpiniae Oxyphyllae), and Wu Bei Zi (Galla Chinensis).

Functions: Nourishing yin, clearing away heat, and inducing astringency.

(9) Xiaoke Ping Fang(Tablets for Treating Diabetes, from *Journal of Shandong College of Traditional Chinese Medicine*; 1985,(5))

Ingredients: Huang Qi(Radix Astragali seu Hedysari), Ren Shen (Radix Ginseng), Tian Hua Fen (Radix Trichosanthis), Zhi Mu (Rhizoma Anemarrhenae), Ge Gen(Radix Puerariae), Tian Dong (Radix Asparagi), Wu Wei Zi(Fructus Schisandrae), Sha Yuan Zi (Semen Astragali Complanati), and Dan Shen(Radix Salviae Miltiorrhizae).

Preparation: Make the above drugs into tablets to be taken 6 — 8 tablets each time, three times daily. One month forms a course of treatment and three courses are necessary. Or the formula may also be taken in the form of decoction.

Functions: Supplementing qi, nourishing yin, and promoting the production of body bluid to quench thirst.

(10) Xiaosanduo Tang (Decoction for Removing Polydipsia, polyphagia and polyuria, from *Henan Traditional Chinese Medicine*; 1987,(5): 33)

Ingredients: Ren Shen (Radix Ginseng), Zhi Mu (Rhizoma Anemarrhenae), Shi Gao (Gypsum Fibrosum), Huang Lian (Rhizoma Coptidis), E Jiao (Colla Corii Asini), Bai Shao (Radix Paeoniae Alba), Tian Hua Fen (Radix Trichosanthis), Shan Yao (Rhizoma Dioscoreae), Huang Jing (Rhizoma Polygonati), Zheng Shou Wu (Radix Polygoni Multiflori Praeparata), Mai Dong (Radix Ophiopogonis), Di Gu Pi(Cortex Lycii Radicis), and Yolk.

Preparation: To be decocted in water for oral dose, one dose daily.

Functions: Nourishing the liver-yin and the kidney-yin, moistening dryness, supplementing qi, clearing away heat, and promoting the production of body fluid to quench thirst.

(11) Qi Shu Huafen Tang (Decoction of Astragalus, Dioscorea

and Trichosanthes, from *Shanghai Journal of Traditional Chinese Medicine*; 1983, (8): 28)

Ingredients: Huang Qi(Radix Astragali seu Hedysari), Shan Yao (Rhizoma Dioscoreae), Sang Bai Pi(Cortex Mori Radicis), Di Gu Pi (Cortex Lycii Radicis), Shi Hu(Herba Dendrobii), and Tian Hua Fen(Radix Trichosanthis).

Preparation: To be decocted in water for oral dose.

Functions: Supplementing qi, nourishing yin, and promoting the production of body fluid to quench thirst.

(12) Huanglian Jiangtang San(Coptis Powder for Reducing Blood Sugar, from *Shandong Journal of Traditional Chinese Medicine*; 1983, (5):15)

Ingredients: Huang Lian(Rhizoma Coptidis), Dang Shen(Radix Codonopsis Pilosulae) or Ren Shen(Radix Ginseng), Tian Hua Fen (Radix Trichosanthis), and Ze Xie(Rhizoma Alismatis).

Preparation: Grind the drugs above together into powder to be taken with warm-boiled water, 3g each time, three times a day.

Functions: Clearing away heat, supplementing qi and nourishing yin.

(13) Qi Yin Guben Tang(Decoction for Strengthening Defensive Qi and Tonifying Yin, from *The Encyclopedia of Proved Prescriptions of Contemporary Famous TCM Doctors in China*)

Ingredients: Huang Qi(Radix Astragali seu Hedysari), Shan Yao (Rhizoma Dioscoreae), Sheng Di (Radix Rehmanniae), Shu Di (Radix Rehmanniae Praeparata), Cang Zhu (Rhizoma Atractylodis), Mai Dong(Radix Ophiopogonis), Wu Wei Zi(Fructus Schisandrae), Wu Bei Zi(Galla Chinensis), Mu Li(Concha Ostreae), Fu Ling(Poria), Tian Hua Fen(Radix Trichosanthis), Ge Gen(Radix Puerariae), and Shan Yu Rou(Fructus Corni).

Preparation: First soak the drugs above in clear water for 30 minutes, then decoct them for 30 minutes twice to be taken in the morning and evening, one dose daily.

Functions: Supplementing qi, nourishing yin, promoting the production of body fluid to quench thirst, astringing essence and consolidating the kidney.

(14) Yiqi Xuanyin Yin(Drink for Supplementing Qi and Nourishing Yin, from *The Encyclopedia of Proved Prescriptions of Contemporary Famous TCM Doctors in China*)

Ingredients: Huang Qi(Radix Astragali seu Hedysari), Ren Shen (Radix Ginseng), Dang Shen(Radix Codonopsis Pilosulae), Yu Zhu (Rhizoma Polygonati Multiflori), Sheng Di(Radix Rehmanniae), Shan Yao(Rhizoma Dioscoreae), Gou Qi Zi(Fructus Lycii), Tian Dong(Radix Asparagi), Tu Si Zi(Semen Cuscutae), Nu Zhen Zi (Fructus Ligustri Lucidi), and Xuan Shen(Radix Scrophulariae).

Preparation: The above drugs are to be soaked in water for 30 minutes, then decocted in the water for 30 minutes twice, to be taken in the morning and evening respectively,one dose daily.

Functions: Supplementing qi and nourishing yin.

(15) Yuxiao Ling(Effective Prescription for Diabetes, from *The Encyclopedia of Proved Prescriptions of Contempory Famous TCM Doctors in China*)

Ingredients: Huang Qi(Radix Astragali seu Hedysari), Shan Yao (Rhizoma Dioscoreae), Huang Jing(Rhizoma Polygonati), Shi Hu (Herba Dendrobii),Hua Fen(Radix Trichosanthis),Sheng Di(Radix Rehmanniae), Shu Di(Radix Rehmanniae Praeparata), Zhu Ye (Lophatherum), Di Gu Pi(Cortex Lycii Radicis),Jiang Can Fen (Bombyx Batryticatus,powdered).

Preparation: Soak the above drugs in water for 30 minutes and decoct them for another 30 minutes twice. Mix the decoctions with each other to be taken twice,one dose daily.

Functions: Nourishing yin, clearing away heat, supplementing qi, promoting the production of the body fluid, astringing qi and consolidating essence.

(16) Sang Mei Qizi Yin(Drink of Seeds of Seven Drugs with Mul-

berry Leaf and Prunus Mume, from *Hebei Traditional Chinese Medicine*, 1987,(5):37)

Ingredients: Sang Ye(Folium Mori), Wu Mei(Fructus Mume), Tu Si Zi(Semen Cuscutae), Fu Pen Zi(Fructus Rubi),Gou Qi Zi (Fructus Lycii), Nu Zhen Zi(Fructus Ligustri Lucidi), Sha Yuan Zi (Semen Astragali Complanati), Wu Bei Zi(Galla Chinensis) and Wu Wei Zi(Fructus Schisandrae).

Preparation: To be decocted in water for oral dose.

Functions: Moderately tonifying both yin and yang, moistening dryness and quenching thirst.

(17) Jiangtong Tang(Decoction for Reducing Ketone, from *Jilin-Traditional Chinese Medicine*,1988;(4):12)

Ingredients: Sheng Huang Qi (Radix Astragali seu Hedysari), Shan Yao(Rhizoma Dioscoreae), Xuan Shen(Radix Scrophulariae), Cang Zhu(Rhizoma Atractylodis), Huang Qin(Radix Scutellariae), Huang Lian(Rhizoma Coptidis), Huang Bai(Cortex Phellodendri), Zhi Zi(Fructus Gardeniae), Sheng Di(Radix Rehmanniae), Dang Gui(Radix Angelicae Sinensis), Chuan Xiong(Rhizoma Ligustici Chuanxiong),Chi Shao(Radix Paeoniae Rubra), Fu Ling(Poria), and Mu Li(Concha Ostreae).

Preparation: To be decocted in water for oral dose, one dose daily.

Functions: Supplementing qi and nourishing yin, and clearing away heat from blood.

4. 3 The commonly-used simple and proved formulas

① Grind equal amount of Tian Hua Fen (Radix Trichosanthis) and Huang Lian (Rhizoma Coptidis) into fine powder to make pills with water. Take the pills with decoction of Mai Men Dong (Radix Ophiopogonis), 3g each time, twice a day.

② Decoct Bu Gu Zhi (Fructus Psoraleae) 15g and Huang Qi (Radix Astragali seu Hedysari Praeparata) 15g, Xiao Hui Xiang

(Fructus Foenicuii, parched with salt) 6g in boiling water and then remove the dregs. Take the decoction every evening.

③ Pork pancreas 1 piece, eggs 3 pieces, and spinach 60g. Slice and then cook the pork pancreas, stir the eggs and cook them with Spinace. Eat and drink them together once a day.

④ Sea cucumber, egg and pork pancreas 1 piece each. Cook and eat them with soy sauce, one dose every other day.

⑤ Zhuyi Shanyao Tang(Decoction of Pork Pancreas and Chinese Yam): Pork Pancreas 1 piece, Shan Yao(Rhizoea Dioscoreae) 60g, to be cooked and taken orally.

⑥ River snail 500g and Water 1500ml. Soak the River snails in the water for one night. Then, cook the snail in the water to be eaten with the soup, one dose daily.

⑦ Parch and grind equal amount of Hei Da Dou(Semen Sojae Nigrum) and Tian Hua Fen(Radix Trichosanthis) into powder, make the powder into pills as big as Chinese Parasol seeds, and take 70 pills with black bean soup each time, twice a day.

⑧ Cook Lu Dou(Semen Phaseoli Radiati), take it orally as congee, or as its soup.

⑨ Pound the radish and drink its juice , or make congee with the juice and eat it.

⑩ Decoct the wax gourd in water. Take 100—150g of the decoction after each meal. This can induce diuresis to alleviate edema.

⑪ Stigma Maydis 30g, decocted in water and taken as tea.

⑫ Cook pork spleen with Chi Xiao Dou(Semen Phaseoli, sprouted better), to be taken orally frequently.

⑬ Decoct Shan Yao(Rhizoma Dioscoreae) in water to something of congee to be taken orally, one medium-sized bowl each time. In autumn and winter buy fresh Chinese yam, cook and eat it. If the fresh one can not be bought, buy it(dried slices) in Chinese drug stores. Grind it into powder and make the powder into paste with boiling water. Then cook it a little while to be taken one small bowl each

115

time.

⑭ Parch silkworm chrysalis to be taken 6g each time, 3 times daily, for 10 days.

⑮ Live clam, to be shelled, pounded and stewed to be taken warm, several times a day.

⑯ Celery 500g, to be ground into juice and boiled or decocted in water for oral dose.

⑰ Zhu Li(Sucus Bambosae) 30-60g, to be decocted in water and then taken freely for several days.

⑱ Decoct Sang Shen (Fructus Mori) into cream to be taken 2 spoons with boiling water in the moring and evening.

⑲ Water spinach 100g and Yu Mi Xu(Stigma Maydis) 50g, to be decocted in water for continuous administration of 7—10 days.

⑳ Green pea, to be decocted and taken without any flavor; or tender pea seedling, to be pounded into juice and taken a half cup each time, twice daily.

㉑ Da Hei Dou (Semen Sojae Nigrum) 50g and Tian Hua Fen (Radix Trichosanthis) 50g, to be decocted in water for oral dose.

㉒ Puffed Nuo Mi(Glutinous Rice) 50g and Sang Bai Pi(Cortex Mori Radicis) 20g, to be decocted in water and taken orally, twice daily.

㉓ Big river snail 10 pieces, to be kept alive in water to make the dirty things out of them, shelled, added a little millet wine, then stirred and stewed in water. Both the soup and the shelled river shails are taken orally once or twice times daily.

㉔ Bai Mao Gen(Rhizoma Imperatae) 60—90g, to be decocted in water, and taken as tea, one dose a day. Ten days continuous administration will cure the disease.

㉕ Fresh root of spinach 90g and Ji Nei Jin(Endothelium Corneum Gigeriae Galli) 15g, to be decocted in water and taken orally, 2—3 times daily.

㉖ Xi Gua Cui Yi(Exocarpium Citrulli) 15g, to be decocted in wa-

116

ter and taken orally, 3 times daily for several days.

㉗ Yuhu Wan(Jade Tiger Pill): equal amount of Tian Hua Fen (Radix Trichosanthis) and Ren Shen(Radix Ginseng), to be ground into powder and made into pills as big as Chinese parasol seeds with honey and then taken 30 pills each time with Maimendong Tang (Ophiopogon Decoction) for quenching thirst, supplementing qi and promoting the production of body fluid.

㉘ Grind Huang Qi(Radix Astragali seu Hedysari) into powder, put it in pig's tripe, and steam it to be tender enough to eat for supplementing qi, clearing away heat and quenching thirst.

㉙ Fresh Ou Zhi(Liquidom Nelumbinis Rhizomatis), to be taken at a draught.

㉚ Zhuji Tang(Decoction of Pork Backbone): Pork backbone segment, 0. 4m long, Da Zao(Fructus Ziziphi Jujubae) 10 pieces, Lian Zi(fresh Semen Nelumbinis) 49 pieces, Gan Cao (Radix Glycyrrhizae Praeparata) 10g, Mu Xiang(Radix Aucklandiae) 15g, and water 5 bowls, to be decocted into one bowl for frequent oral use.

㉛ Shan Yao(Rhizoma Dioscoreae) 250g and Hua Fen(Radix Trichosanthis) 250g, to be parched a little, ground into powder, mixed up evenly, and then divided into 30 packs. One pack is taken daily with boiled water.

㉜ For diabetes with irritability, decoct dry pulp of wax gourd 30g in water for oral dose.

㉝ For thirst and turbid urine, decoct Xi Gua Pi(Exocarpium Citrulli) 15g, Dong Gua Pi(Exocarpium Benincasae) 15g and Tian Hua Fen(Radix Trichosanthis) 15—20g in water for oral dose.

㉞ For diabetes with obesity: Huang Jing(Rhizoma Polygonati) 15g, Ze Xie(Rhizoma Alismatis) 15g, He Ye(Folium Nelumbinis) 15g, Hu Zhang(Rhizoma Polygoni Cuspidati) 15g, and Shan Zha (Fructus Crataegi) 15g, to be decocted in water and taken orally, once a day.

117

㉟ Equal amount of Rou Cong Rong(Herba Cistanchis), Shan Yu Rou (Fructus Corni), and Wu Wei Zi(Fructus Schisandrae), to be ground together into powder, and made into pills as big as Chinese parasol seeds with water. 20 pills are taken each time.

㊱ Fresh Ma Chi Xian(Herba Potulacae) 30g, to be decocted in water and taken as tea together with the drug. This can clear away heat and remove toxic materials.

㊲ Ju Hua(Flos Chrysanthemi), moderate amount, to be infused with boiling water and taken as tea for removing intensive heat from the liver and improving acuity of sight.

㊳ Tu Si Zi (Semen Cuscutae), to be decocted to get the juice which is to be taken freely for nourishing the kidney and essence.

㊴ Ji Cai(Herba Capsellae), to be scalded with boiling water, and then cooled and dressed with sauce for eating to clear away heat, detoxicate and reduce the blood pressure.

Chapter 5   Diabetes in the Aged

With the development of the medical science, many commonly seen infectious diseases and parasitosis in the past have been gradually eliminated or controlled. And the average life span of the human kind has been prolonged by degrees. Gerontology will become a major topic of the future medicine. During the investigation of diabetes among 100 000 populations in Shanghai in 1978, it was found that the incidence of the disease in the aged has a tendency to increase together with the age. After 40 years old, the incidence of the disease increases rapidly in both males and females, reaching its peak at the age from 60 to 70. And it is four times that of the whole populations. This shows that diabetes is a common and frequently seen disease in the aged. The results of the reports both at home and abroad are fundamentally the same, indicating the above mentioned is a universal phenomena. Diabetes will become a major commonly seen disease in the future with the improvement of the economic and living conditions. Thus, prevention and treatment of the disease is a concerned topic in modern medical field.

The senile diabetes generally refers to that occurring in the population over 60 years old. As a result of the invention of insulin and the wide application of antibiotics, the sum of the cases complicated by or dying of infections or ketoacidosis has been reduced remarkably, and the life span of the patients has been obviously prolonged. Most of the patients may live to the senile age through proper treatment. Therefore, diabetes of the aged includes two kinds: the diabetes occurring after 60 years old and the diabetes occurring before 60 years old but still existing over 60 years old. the morbidity of the disease grows with the age, and rises rapidly in the population from 40 to 50 years old. Almostly it increases by 10% per 10 year after 40, and reaches its highest peak at the age of 70. The total morbidity of the disease at the age of 70 is about three times that of the whole populations and the disease affects mainly the females. This showes that diabetes is really a common and frequently seen disease in the aged. With the constant improvement of the living conditions, the life apan will be gradually prolonged, and the old people will become more and more. So, senile diabetes, which may be more easily complicated by cardiocerebrovascular or nervous disorders, will be more commonly seen and become a major life-threatening disease of the aged, and the prevention and treatment of it appear to be more important.

5. 1 Prevention and Treatment of Senile Diabetes

5. 1. 1 Educational Propaganda

Provide constant routine education for the diabetics and this demand is never too excessive. In the propaganda, special emphasis should be palced on the prevention of hypertonics (avoidance of eating sweat food), diabetic feet and avoidance of burn, injury and infection.

5. 1. 2 Diet-control

Except for the general requirment, the patient's favorite should be considered in order to acquire his or her cooperation. Food with high sugar or more fibers, which is a popular schedule for diabetics diet at aboard, is also available in China, as it is simple and practical. According to this schedule, colories contained in the sugar should be 60% of the total calories consumed, and more than 15mg of fibers should be given per day.

5. 1. 3 Physical exercise

Physical exercise should be encouraged, but before the exercise, such contraindications as acute or chronic complications of the disease should be noticed, and the functions of the heart and the lung should be well evaluated.

Diet-control and proper physical exercise are the basis of treatment of the senile diabetes for the purpose of improving the glucometabolism. If this method can not control the disease, medications should be given.

5. 1. 4 Medications

Oral antihyperglykemic should be the key medicine for senile diabetes. Insulin cannot be administered unless there is no alternation. As the seniles are very sensitive to antihyperglycemic, the drug should be administered in a strictly confined dosage or under the guide of the doctors, otherwise cardiac infarct or cerebrovascular disorders may occasionally follow, which will affect the patient's health severely. And as the etiology of the disease is still not well known, the oral use of antihyperglycemic aims only at the relief of hyperglucose, or the treatment of symptoms with reducing sugar as its core. So it is not an accomplished therapy because it cannot erase the cause of the disease. Today, diabetes, which falls into the categoey of Xiaoke Syndrome in TCM, is being widely treated with herbal medicine in accordance with its different types of syndromes. This suggests that only the treatment is based on the different syndromes can the senile diabetes be cured by erasing its basic cause.

5. 2 TCM Treatment of Senile Diabets

5. 2. 1 Etiology and Pathogenesis

Diabetes in the aged is mainly caused by decline of the vital qi and weakness of the five zang organs, especially the weakness of the spleen and stomach. In case of improper diet, emotional stimuli and sexual incontinence, the disease may be induced. Long-standing improper diet, or excessive intake of sweat and fatty food and over intake of alcohol, may impair the spleen-qi, leading to failure of the spleen to lift nutrients and the production of internal heat, which in turn, consumes body fluid and leads to hyperactive digestion. Prolonged emotional stimuli may cause disturbance of the liver, transverse attack of the liver on the spleen and stomach, and the heat transformed from the stagnated qi, leading to injury of the yin-fluid of the lung and the stomach. Original yin-deficiency together with sexual incontinence may consumes the kidney-essence, leading to failure of the kidney to store essence and control opening and closing, or leadingg to hyperactivity of the ministerial fire and the further impairment of yin-fluid. Of these different pathological changes, the common point is the impairment of yin by interior heat. Therefore, the fundamental pathogenesis of the disease lies in yin deficiency and dryness-heat with the former as its foundation. In a prolonged case, deficiency of both qi and yin may present as a result of the consumption of yin and qi, which may further involves yang and lead to deficiency of both yin and yang at the later stage of the disease. Prolonged qi deficiency, yin deficiency or stagnation of fire may cause blood stasis in the vessels, leading to various complicated morbid conditions and accompanying manifestations.

TCM believes that when one reaches the old age, there are weakness of zang-fu organs, imbalance between yin and yang, insufficiency of qi and blood, blood stasis and general weakness. As a result, the functional activities of the body declines. The results of the study in both ancient and modern times all indicate that the main reasons of aging are spleen-deficiency and kidney-deficiency, which are the most commonly seen syndomes in the deficiency syndromes of the aged. In addition, signs of blood stasis are also very popular in the aged because of their deficient qi and blood often leading to sluggish or impeded flow of the blood. So besides the dryness-heat due to yin deiciency, kidney deficiency, deficiency of both the spleen and stomach and obstruction of blood in the vessels should also be noticed. To sum up, senile diabetes in fact originates from deficiency of both the spleen and the kidney, and is manifested as dryness-heat and blood stasis. The kidney and the spleen, which are regarded as the source of the congenital genuine qi and the source of the qi and blood after

122

birth respectively, assist each other, thereby promoting the growth and development of the body and the production of qi, blood and body fluid. If one is strong in both qi and mental activities and rich in essence and blood, he or her will not suffer from disease, whereas if his or her spleen-qi is weak and fails to transform and transport, the kidney will lose the supplement of nutrients from the spleen, leading to deficiency of the kidney-essence and the ensuing hypofunction of the kidney. So the spleen and the kidney also influence each other pathologically, and there is a relationship of mutual reason and result. This is why deficiency of the spleen and kidney often occurs simultaneously. To be exact, the senile diabetes often appears as the result of the weakness of both the spleen and kidney due to aging.

5. 2. 2 Syndrome identification and treatment

As the pathogenesis of the senile diabetes is rather complicated, involving disorders of yin and yang, qi and blood and zang-fu organs, especially the hypofunction of the spleen and the kidney and the insufficiency of the pectorial qi, syndrome of qi deficiency and blood stasis are usually seen. As the disease in the aged has a slow onset and is often accompanied with secondary syndromes or complications, it is hard to be controlled in a short time. And as it is a chronic disease, often a life-long disease, application of western medicine usually can not bring about remarkably effect. On the other hand, if herbal medicine can be applied on the basis of diet-control, physical exercise and western medicine, satisfactory therapeutic effects can be expected to achieve. This is because TCM treatment is aimed at the regulation of the whole body and the treatment of the fundamental cause of the disease in light of the syndromes identification. TCM treatment can not only relieve the symptoms, but also help to restore strength and reduce the side or adverse effects of the oral antihypemecia. Of course, TCM treatment should be carried out based on the treatment of Xiaoke in TCM.

1) Kiney deficiency as the main syndrome

Main manifestations: dizziness, tinnitus, soreness and weakness of the loins, blurring of vision, tidal fever, night sweat, loose teeth and fall of hair, increased nocturnal urine, impotence, pale tongue with thin and whitish or little coating, deep thready or thready wiry pulse.

Kidney deficiency mainly refers to the deficiency of essence stored in the kidney. The kidney, which is regarded as the basis of the congenital constitution of the body, stores essence that contains the genuine yin and genuine yang, dominates water metabolism and receives the nutrients from other zang organs. So it serves as the basis of the premorial qi and the five zang organs, and the essence of it works as the fundamental force of the functional activities of the body. This is what is called "the kidney, an organ controlling water metabolism, dominates the body fluid", or "water connects with the kidney". The kidney essence exerts its physiological effects in two ways, kidney yin and kidney yang. The former refers to the effects of nourishing and moistening zang fu organs and other parts of the body, while the latter, the effects of warming and impulsing. In normal conditions, the kidney yin and kidney yang supply and restrict each other. When the kidney essence is deficient, the kidney yin and kidney yang will also be deficient, and the kidney will thus lose the function of controlling water metabolism, giving rise to abnormal distribution and discharge of the body fluid and the resultant occurrence of the diabetes. As the body fluid fails to be steamed upward, there is polydipsia, as the essence fails to be stored, there is sweat urine, and as the opening and closing of the bladder fails to be controlled, there is polyuria. All the above suggests that kidney deficinecy is an important factor contributing to the disease.

Therapeutic method: tonifying the kidney, supported by activating flow of the blood.

Prescription: Shan Yao(Rhizoma Dioscoreae) 15g, Shan Yu Rou (Fructus Corni) 15g, Sheng Di Huang(Radix Rehmanniae) 15g,

124

Gou Qi Zi(Fructus Lycii) 15g, Ge Gen(Radix Puerariae) 15g, Chi Shao(Radix Paeoniae Rubra)15g, Ze Xie(Rhizoma Alismatis) 15g, Shu Di(Radix Rehmanniae Praeparata) 12g, Sha Yuan Zi(Semen Astragali Complatanati) 30g, He Shou Wu(Radix Polygoni Multiflori) 30g, Huang Qi(Radix Astragali seu Hedysari) 30g, Hua Fen (Radix Trichosanthis) 30g, Dan Shen(Radix Salviae Miltiorrhizae) 30g, Di Gu Pi(Cortex Lycii Radicis) 20g.

The above herbs are to be decocted in water for oral use.

In this formula, Shan Yao, Shan Yu Rou, Sheng Di Huang, Gou Qi Zi, Sha Yuan Zi and He Shou Wu are used to nourish the kidney Yin, Hua Fen, Ge Gen, Di Gu Pi and Ze Xie, to clear away heat and promote the production of the body fluid to relieve thirst, Huang Qi to strengthen the spleen qi to tonify the kidney, and Chi Shao and Dan Shen to activate blood flow and remove blood stasis.

Modern pharmacological research shows that He Shou Wu and Ze Xie can lower the blood pressure and the cholesterol and thus are the best herbs for senile diabetes with hyperlipemia and arteriosclerosis. This formula is mainly aimed at nourishing the kidney yin by the asistance of clearing away heat, promoting the production of the body fluid, activating the blood flow and removing blood stasis. It can be used to lower the blood pressure, hyperlipemia, blood sugar and urine glucose, and is especially suitable for the aged.

Modifications:

① In the case of incompletely relieved dryness-heat, which is manifested as dry mouth and tongue, irritability, dark urine, constipation, red tongue with little coating,the treatment should be still directed at nourishing yin and moistening the lung, clearing away lung heat and promoting the production of the body fluid. Sheng Shi Gao (Gypsum Fibrum), Zhi Mu(Rhizoma Anemarrhenae), Sha Shen (Radix Adenophorae Strictae), Mai Dong (Radix Ophiopogonis), Xuan Shen(Radix Scrophulariae), Huang Lian(Radix Coptis) and Large amount of Hua Fen should be added to the above formula. Or,

Bai Hu Jia Ren Shen Tang (White Tiger Decoction with Radix Ginseng) or Xiao Ke Fang is administered first, which is replaced by the formula tonifying the kidney when it is effective.

② In the case of obvious qi deficiency, marked by lassitude, shortness of breath and disinclination to talk, tender and enlarged tongue with thin and whitish coating, weak and forceless pulse, the dosage of Huang Qi should be increased and Ren Shen (Radix Ginseng) and Dang Shen (Radix Codonopsis Pilosulae) added.

③ In the case of frequency of nocturnal urine or incontinence of urine, Fu Pen Zi (Fructus Rubi), Wu Bei Zi (Galla Sinensis), Yi Zhi Ren (Fructus Alpiniae Oxyphyllae) and Sang Piao Xiao (Oothec Mantidis) are to be added.

④ In the case of abdominal distension and hypochondriac pain, Chuan Lian Zi (Fructus Meliae Toosendan) and Li Zhi He (Semen Litchi) are to be added.

⑤ In the case of loose stool or diarrhea, Bai Zhu (Rhizoma Atractylodis Macrocepgalae), Fu Ling (Poria), and Yi Yi Ren (Semen Coicis) are to be added and the yin-nourishing drugs in the formula such as Sheng Di Huang reduced.

⑥ In the case of severe deficiency of the kidney-Yang, Tu Si Zi (Semen Trigonellae), Hu Lu Ba (Semen Trigomellae), and Xian Ling Pi (Herba Epimedii) are to be added.

⑦ In the case of numbness of limbs, Quan Xie (Scorpio), Wu Gong (Scolopendra), Di Long (Lumbricus) and Ji Xie Teng (Caulis Millettiae) are to be added, if there is also gangrene of the limbs, dosage of the drugs invigorating qi and activating blood flow in the formula should be increased and those warming up yang-qi to promote blood flow should be added in accordance with the patients' conditions.

⑧ If the disease is mainly manifested as blood stasis and complicated by cardiocerebrovascular diseases, invigorating qi to promote the flow of blood should be the chief method of treatment.

⑨ In the case of hectic fever, Da Bu Yin Wan (Bolus with A Strong Action of Nourishing Yin) is to be used together with the formula, or Zhi Mu (Rhizoma Anemarrheae) and Huang Bai (Cortex Phellodendri) are to be added to it.

2) Qi deficiency as the main syndrome

Main manifestations: Obesity, lassitude, oppressed feeling in the chest, shortness of breath, lassitude, spontaneous sweating or night sweating, lustreless face, no obvious polyphagia, polydipsia, polyuria and loss of weight, moderate elevation of blood glucose, pale and enlarged tongue with teeth prints on its margin, and thready weak pulse.

These symptoms and signs are ascribed to failure of the qi and blood to be moved due to decline of the primordial qi of the aged and the ensuing insufficient function of the heart and the lung, and the hypofunction of the spleen and stomach which leads to decreased digestion and insufficient source of the nutrients. These two aspects will finally cause deficiency of the zang-fu organs, obstruction of defensive qi and nutritive qi and the formation of diabetes. As for the role of the vital qi in the occurrence of diabetes, decline of the pectorial qi is an original cause; as for the role of pathogens, the disease is induced by the stagnated heat in the lung and the spleen and the stomach fire, which consumes both the body fluid and the primordial qi. Therefore, the routine treatment for diabetes is to tonify qi, nourish yin and clear away heat.

Therapeutic method: Tonifying qi, nourishing yin and clearing away heat.

Prescription: Huang Qi (Radix Astragali seu Hedysari) 30g, Ren Shen (Radix Ginseng) 15g, Shan Yao (Rhizoma Dioscoreae) 15g, Bai Shao 15g, Shan Yu Rou (Fructus Corni) 15g, Ge Gen (Radix Puerariae) 15g, Mai Dong (Radix Ophiopogonis) 12g, Wu Wei Zi (Fructus Schisandrae) 10g, Zhi Mu (Rhizoma Aemarrhenae) 10g, Sheng Ma (Rhizoma Cimicifugae) 6g, Chai Hu (Radix Bulpleuri) 6g, Cang

127

Zhu(Rhizoma Atractylodis) 18g, Xuan Shen(Radix Scrophulariae) 12g, Dan Shen (Radix Salviae Miltiorrhizae) 30g, and Sang Ji Sheng(Ramulus Loranthis) 15g.

The above drugs are to be decocted in water for oral dose.

In this formula, Huang Qi and Ren Shen are used as the main drugs to tonify qi; Shan Yao to nourish both the spleen yin and the kidney yin; and Cang Zhu to promote the transforming and transporting action of the spleen yang. As Cang Zhu is dry in nature, Xuan Shen is administered in this formula to restrict the dryness of Cang Zhu. These two drugs are often used together to promote the function of the spleen yang to decrease blood sugar and have been proved highly effective for diabetes with a strong effect of decreasing the blood sugar. Besides, Shan Yu Rou is used to tonify the kidney and the liver to prevent exhaustion of the primordial qi; Sheng Ma and Chai Hu to lift qi; Mai Dong to nourish the lung yin; Wu Wei Zi to astringe the lung qi; Zhi Mu to clear away heat and moisten dryness; Bai Shao to nourish the liver blood; Ge Gen to relieve thirst by promoting the production of body fluid and induce the body fluid to go upward by lifting the lucid yang of the spleen and the stomach; and Sang Ji Sheng, combined with Huang Qi, to tonify qi and fortify the kidney. This formula is derived from Sheng Xian Tang (Decoction for Treating Collapse of the Pectoral Qi), a formula advanced by Mr. Zhang Xichun. It is indicative for collapse of the pectoral qi marked by shortness of breath, dry mouth and thirst. Satisfactory effects have been achieved in the treatment of 60 cases of diabetes with modified Sheng Xian Tang in Shandong Traditional Chinese Medicine hospital.

Modifications:

① For cases of deficiency of both qi and yin-fluid, marked by dry mouth and throat, lassitude, disinclination to talk, red tongue with little coating, and thready and rapid pulse, the therapeutic method should be aimed at tonifying qi and nourishing yin by adopting Sheng

128

Mai San (Pulse Activating Powder) in combination with Liu Wei Di Huang Tang (Decoction of Six Drugs with Rhizoma Rehmanniae Praeparata), or Huang Qi Tang(Radix Astragali seu Hedysari Decoction) in combination with Yu Ye Tang(Decoction for Nourishing Precious Fluid), etc.

② For cases of deficiency of both yin and yang due to the lingering deficient yin affecting yang, marked by frenquent turbid urine with large volume, or polyuria at night, aversion to cold, cold limbs, or even impotence, diarrhea, and edema, the treatment should be directed at tonifying both yin and yang and regulating both qi and blood. Such formulas as Jin Kui Shen Qi Wan(Kidney-Qi Invigorating Pill) and You Gui Yin(Kidney-Yang Reinforcing Decoction) can be selected. To these formulas, Yang Qi Shi(Actinolitum) and Xian Ling Pi(Herba Epimedii) should be added in the case of impotence; and Bai Zhu(Rhizoma Atractylodis Macrocephalae), Yi Mi(Semen Coicis), Bu Gu Zhi(Fructus Psoraleae) and Mi Qiao(Rice Shell) in the case of diarrhea. In the case of edema, Ji Sheng Shen Qi Wan (Life Preserving Pill for Supplementing the Kidney-Qi), to which Yi Mu Cao(Herba Leonuri)and Yu Mi Xu(Stigma Maydis), and the drugs activating blood flow by removing blood stasis such as Dan Shen (Radix Salviae Miltiorrhizae), Chi Shao (Radix Paeonia Rubra), and Ze Lan(Herba Lycopi)are added, can be administered.

3) Retention of dampness due to deficiency of the spleen-qi

Main manifestations: thirst but not desire for drinking, dry mouth with sticky and greasy taste, dizziness, headache, heaviness of the body, epigastriac and abdominal fullness, poor appetite, loose stool, pale and enlarged tongue proper with thick and greasy coating, and moderate and slow pulse.

This syndrome arise from over intake of fat and spicy foods, which leads to production of damp-heat in the spleen and stomach and the ensuing abnormality of Qi's activities.

Therapeutic method: Strengthening the spleen to eliminate dampness, assisted by clearing away the stomach-heat.

Prescription: Dang Shen (Radix Codonopsis Pilosulae) 15g, Fu Ling (Poria) 15g, Ge Gen (Radix Puerariae) 15g, Yi Mi (Semen Coicis) 15g, Bai Bian Dou (Semen Dolichoris Album) 15g, Bai Zhu (Radix atrctylodis Macrocephalae) 12g, Mu Xiang (Radix Aucklandiae) 9g, Huo Xiang (Herba Agastachis) 9g, Shan Yao (Rhioma Dioscoreae) 12g, Bai Kou Ren (Semen Amomi Cardamomi) 10g, and Gan Cao (Radix Glycirrhizae) 6g.

The above drugs are to be decocted in water for oral use.

In this formula, Dang Shen, Fu Ling, Bai Zhu and Gan Cao (the four drugs of the Decoction of the Four Noble Drugs) are used to strengthen the spleen and benefit qi; Ge Gen to promote production of the body fluid to quench thirst; Mu Xiang to promote flow of qi; Huo Xiang, aromatic in taste, to dissolve turbid dampness; Shan Yao, Yi Mi, Bian Dou, Sha Ren and Bai Kou to revive the spleen to eliminate dampness. In the treatment of diabetes, the purpose of strengthening the spleen is to promote the production of the body fluid and control qi. Therefore, drugs bland in taste should be adopted to nourish the stomach, lift the lucid and benefit Qi. Be sure not to apply the drugs bitter in taste and dry in nature. In addition, drugs sour and sweet in tastes, such as Wu Mei (Fructus Mume), Wu Wei Zi (Fructus Schisandrae), Ren Shen (Radix Ginseng), Mai Dong (Radix Ophiopogonis), Hua Fen (Radix Trichosanthis) and Di Huang (Radix Rehmanniae), can be added to nourish yin, regulate yin and yang and promote the production of body fluid, according to patients' conditions.

Modifications:

① In the case of stomach heat accompanied with dampness and the disturbed distribution of body fluid and qi, marked by dry mouth, emaciation with polyphagia, spontaneous sweating, thirst with preference for drinks, dry stool, frequent urination, red tongue with greasy coating, soft and rapid pulse, Lan Xiang Yin Zi (Lan Xiang Decoction) with modifications should be administered to purge the stomach heat, regulate flow of qi in the middle jiao and lift body fluid.

② For cases with severe oppressed feeling in the epigastrium and abdomen; add Chen Pi (Pericarpium Citri Reticulatae), Chai Hu (Radix Bupleuri)and Fo Shou(Fructus Citri Sarcodacltylis).

③ If the patients are complicated by hyperlipemia, drugs with blood-lipid-lowering effect, such as Shan Zha(Fructus Crataegi), Ze Xie (Rhizoma Alismatis), Hu Zhang(Rhizoma Polygoni Cuspidati), Cao Jue Ming (Semen Cassiae) and He Ye(Exocarpium Nelumbinis) can be added deliberately.

④ For patients complicated with edema, formulas such as Shi Pi Yin (Decoction for Invigorating the Spleen Yang)should be adopted instead of the above formulas. If the above formulas are to be adopted, they should be added with Ze Lan(Herba Lycopi), Ze Xie(Rhizoma Alismatis), Dong Gua Pi(Exocarpium Benincasae), Che Qian Zi(Semen Plantaginis)and Yi Mu Cao (Herba Leonuri).

⑤ If hepatitis with high transaminase is complicated, Yin Chen (Artemisiae Scopariae), Tu Fu Ling (Rhizoma Smilacis Glabrae), Ban Lan Gen(Radix Istidis), Pu Gong Ying (Herba Taraxic)are to be added. If there is also jaundice, Huang Qin(Radix Scutellariae), Yin Chen(Artemisiae Scopariae) and Da Huang (Radix et Rhizoma Rhei)should be added.

⑥ In the cases complicated by insomnia with restlessness or sensation of crampling of insect or ants in the skin, which are caused by phlegm-heat transformed from retained food in the gastrointestinal tract disturbing upward along meridians, as stated in the chapter of *Notes and Discussion of Conversion of Plain Questions*, "Disorders of the stomach lead to insomnia", the treatment should be aimed at dissolving phlegm, clearing away heat, regulating the function of the stomach and calming the mind with Huang Lian Wen Dan Tang(Coptis Decoction for Clearing Gallbladder Heat) should be employed to eliminate phlegm and heat.

In addition, there are still some important and common syndromes seen in the senile diabetics. For example, blood stasis may be seen in any of the sydromes of diabetes, which is an important agent contributing to the secondary coronary heart disease, angina pectoris or hemiplegia. For such cases, combined use of Bu Yang Huan Wu Tang (Decoction for Recuperating Yang) or Tao He Cheng Qi Tang (Semen Persicae Decoction for Purgation) with Sheng Main San (Pulse-Activating Powder) is of choice to supplementing qi and activate flow of blood. In the case of numbness and pain of limbs, Quan Chong (Buthidae), Di Long (Lumbricus). Shui Zhi (Hirudo) and Ji Xue Teng (Caulis Spatholobi) can be added; and in the case of chest pain or oppressed feeling in the chest, Gua Lou (Fructus Trichosanthis), Yu Jin (Radix Curcumae) and Xie Bai (Bulbus Allii Macrostemi), etc. , can be added deliberatedly.

5. 3 Case Study

Case 1.

Sun is a 65 year-old male retired cadre who came to the hospital and complained of intense thirst with desire for drinking, polyphagia, blurred vision, numbness of limbs and emaciation for more than six months caused by overexertion.

Interrogation: severe thirst, polydipsia, polyphagia, polyuria, blurred vision, numbness of limbs, spontaneous sweating, occasional night sweat, insomnia, dream-disturbed sleep, and cnstipatin.

Inspection: Aged male with consciousness, ruddy skin, dark red tongue with little coating.

Palpation: Deep and thready pulse.

Physical examination: Body weight 75kg, blood pressure, 17. 9/9. 3kPa, normal thyroid, heart rate 70 beats per minute with normal rhythm, arteriosclerosis at both optical fundus. Laboratory test: HB 110 mg/L, WBC, 8. 2×10^9/L, cholesterol, 5. 7mmol/L, triglycerides, 1. 11-6. 11mmol/L, urea nitrogen, 4. 6 mmol/L, blood sugar, 11. 8mmol/L, urine glucose(+++), and urine glucose quanlitative test for 24 hours, 20 grams.

Diagnosis: Xiao Ke Disease(deficiency of both the spleen and the kidney)in light of TCM;Diabetes(insulin-independent, moderate level)in light of Western medicine.

Therapeutic method: Supplementing qi, strengthening the spleen and tonifying the kidney, assisted by activating circulation of blood and removing blood stasis.

Prescription:

① Huang Qi(Radix Astragali seu Hedysari) 30g, Dan Shen(Radix Salviae Miltiorrhizae) 30g, Hua Fen (Radix Trichosanthis) 30g, Shan Yao (Rhizoma Dioscoreae) 15g, Shan Yu Rou (Fructus Cornii) 15g, Gou Qi Zi(Fructus Lycii) 15g, Dang Shen(Radix Codnpsis Pilsulae) 15g, Ge Gen(Radix Puerariae) 15g, Chi Shao(Radix Poaeniae Rubra) 15g, Cang Zhu (Rhizma Atractylodis) 20g, Bai Zhu(Rhizma Atractylodis) 12g,Huang Lian(Rhizoma Coptidis) 6g, Gan Cao(Radix Glycyrrhizae) 6g.

The above drugs are to be decocted in water for oral dose.

② Xiaoke Ping, a patent Chinese drugs, 8 pills each time, three times daily.

③ Glybenzcyclamide, 2. 5 g each time, twice daily, taken before meal.

Reexamination one month later showed that the blood sugar was 8. 8 mmol/L and the urine sugar was (+). He felt great improvement and still had occasional restlessness with feverish sensation and numbness of limbs. So he was prescribed the original formula with Ji Xue Teng (Caulis Mille tiae Reliculatae) 30g added for one more month use. Examination after that indicated the blood sugar was 7. 2mmol/L and the fasting urine sugar negative. But the urine sugar was still + to ++ after meal. Then the above formula was stopped but the oral use of Xiaoke Ping(Tablets for Treating Diabetes), to be taken 8 tablets each time, three times daily, and glybenzcyclamide to

133

be taken one tablet in the morning, were continued to keep the disease stable. Reexamination made every two to three days showed that the blood sugar had been kept around 7—6 mmol/L.

This patient had a short course of the disease and presented no evident complications, so a better therapeutic effect had been obtained. Decoction of Chinese herbs combined with small dose of oral anti-hyperglecemic can quickly lower the blood sugar, but when the blood sugar and the urine sugar were basically controlled, the decoction can be replaced by Chinese patent drugs to reduce the patients economic burden. In most cases, the symptoms of the disease can be cotrolled two months later after a well-controlled diet and application of decoction of Chinese herbs in patients at the early stage. However, to maintain the blood sugar normal, it is imperative for the patients to keep on taking Chinese patent drugs and small dose of Western medicine, otherwise the blood sugar may elevate again.

Case 2.

Cong was a 61-year old retired cadre who had been ill with diabetes for seven years. Admission number: 56563.

The patient had been ill with diabetes with dry mouth, polydipsia, polyphagia, polyuria and emaciation which did not response to the Western drugs such as glyburide and Diamicron. She experienced frequent reattack of the disease and her symptoms were worsened in the past half a month. She was found to have a blood sugar of 14. 5mmol/L and a urine sugar of(＋＋＋＋) in the out-patient section and then was admitted into the hospital after the diagnosis was confirmed. Her presenting manifestations included dry mouth, severe thirst, emaciation, accompanied by lassitude, numbness of limbs, soreness and weakness of loins and knees, blurred vision, profuse sweating, dry stool, red tongue with thin and yellowish coating and deep thready and weak pulse. The blood sugar was 14. 2mmol/L, and the urine ＋＋＋, but the ketone in the urine was not found. The blood-lipid was 6. 5mmol/L and the triglyceride 1. 6mmol/L.

134

Diagnosis: diabetes (non-insulin-dependent type) in the term of Western medicine.

Type identification: deficiency of both qi and yin, and deficiency of both the liver and the kidney.

Prescription: Huang Qi(Radix Astragali seu Hedysari) 30g, Shan Yao (Rhizoma Dioscoreae) 30g, Hua Fen (Radix Trichosanthis) 30g, Sheng Di(Radix Rehmanniae) 15g, Gou Qi Zi(Fructus Lycii) 15g, Ju Hua(Flos Chrysanthemi) 10g, Dan Shen(Radix Salviae Miltiorrhizae) 30g, Wu Wei Zi(Fructus Schsandrae) 9g, Shan Yu Rou (Fructus Corni) 15g, Zhi Mu(Rhizoma Anemarrhenae) 12g, Cang Zhu(Rhizoma Atractylodis) 15g, Xuan Shen(Radix Scrophulariae), Sha Yuan Zi(Semen Astragali Complannati) 30g, Ge Gen(Radix Puerariae) 15g, to be decocted in water for oral use, one dose daily.

After 30 doses of the above formula were used, dry month and other symptoms were greatly relieved, the fasting blood sugar was 9.5mmol/L and the urine sugar +++. After more 30 doses of the formula with proper modifications were administered, the blood sugar was tested 7.2mmol/L and the urine sugar became negative. Then the decoction was stopped and she was instructed to take Xiaoke Wan (Pill for Treating Diabetes), Xiaoke Ping(Tablets for Treating Diabetes) and Liuwei Dihuang Wan(Bolus Containing Six Noble Drugs) to fortify the therapeutic effect.

Chapter 6   Diagnosis and Treatment
of Gravidic Diabetes

With the increasing improvement of the medical conditions, diabetes has become a common diseases related to pregnancy. Gravidic diabete is of two types, the diabetes that occurs during pregnancy, and the diabetes complicated by pregnancy. Both of them are very harmful to the mother and the fetus and cause high incidence of morbidity to the mother and fetus so far, to which special attentions must be paid. Permeating the plancenta easily, oral anti-hyperglycemic sulfaurca permeates may cause hypoglycemia and teras, so they are not suggested. Insuline cannot be used as a routine treatment also. However, TCM treatment can control the diabetes, brings no harm to both the mother and the fetus, thus it should be widely applied.

According to TCM, functional disturbance often occurs in women because of their specific physiological changes concerning menstruation, pregnancy, delivery and glactation. As a result of the impairment of the spleen and the stomach by improper diet, interior heat and consumption of yin fluid may induce the occurrence of diabete in pregnancy. If a pregnant woman has already diabetes before her pregancy, the disease is often aggravated during the pregnancy. This is because that yin blood rushes to the Chong and Ren meridians to nourish the fetus and so it becomes more deficient during the pregnancy, which will cause impairment of qi and blood of zang fu organs and the Chong and Ren meridians. In severe cases, the pregnancy has to be stopped. TCM treatment is indicated in the case of morning sickness marked by nausea, vomiting in the early period, and deficiency of both qi and blood after delivery. Nausea, vomiting accompanied with dizziness and no appetite, or vomiting right after eating, is

136

known as E Zu (morning sickness) in TCM, which is caused by upward attack of the qi from the Chong Meridian and the ensuing disharmony between the liver and the spleen. It may also be caused by the original deficiency of the spleen and stomach, which induces the stomach qi to flow upward. The treatment of gravidic diabetes should be aimed at regulating the function of the middle jiao, suppressing the upward adverse flow of qi to stop vomiting.

6. 1 Syndrome identifiation and corresponding
       treatment of gravidic diabetes

1) Deficiency of the spleen and stomach

Main manifestations: Nausea, vomiting, loss of appetite, bland taste in the mouth or vomiting watery fluid, listlessness, desire for sleep, pale tongue with whitish and moist coating, soft, slippery and forceless pulse. The symptoms of diabetes may not be obvious, and the urine sugar may be less than before due to decrease intake of food.

As a result of the upward attack of qi from the Chong Meridian, the stomach qi fails to go down, instead, it goes adversely upward together with the rushing qi from the Chong Meridian. So vomiting right after eating occurs. Because the deficient yang qi of the middle jiao due to deficiency of both the spleen and the stomach fails to ascend, the turbid qi cannot be lowered and fluid goes up to cause vomiting watery fluid.

Therapeutic method: Strengthening the spleen and regulating the function of the stomach, lowering the upward adverse flow of qi to stop vomiting.

Prescription: Xiang Sha Liujunzi Tang (Decoction of Six Noble Drugs with Aucklandia and Amomi Fruit, from *Treatise on Formulas of Famous Doctors*) with modifications.

Dang Shen (Radix Codonopsis Pilosulae) 15g, Fu Ling (Poria) 15g, Bai Zhu (Rhizoma Atractylodis Macrocephalae) 12g, Ban Xia

(Rhizoma Pinelliae) 10g, Chen Pi(Pericarpium Citri Reticulatae) 9g, Mu Xiang (Radix Aucklandiae) 9g, Sha Ren(Fructus Amomi) 9g, Sheng Jiang(Rhizoma Zingiberis Recens) 9g, Da Zao(Fructus Ziziphi Jujubae) 9g and Gan Cao(Radix Glycyrrhizae) 6g, to be decocted in water for oral dose.

In the prescription, Dang Shen, Bai Zhu, Fu Ling and Gan Cao are used to strengthen the spleen and regulate the function of the stomach; Sha Ren, Sheng Jiang and Ban Xia to warm the stomach, lower the adverse flow of the stomach qi and stop vomiting; and Chen Pi and Mu Xiang to regulate the flow of qi to relieve the stagnation of qi.

2) Disharmony between the liver and the spleen

Main manifestations: vomiting of sour fluid or bitter fluid, fullness and pain in the hypochondriac region, eructation, stenagma, dizziness, distending pain of the head, dysphoria, bitter taste in the mouth, light red tongue with yellowish coating, slippery and wiry pulse. These symptoms occur in the pregnancy and changes in accordance with emotional changes. The manifestations of diabetes are not obvious.

Vomiting is caused by the transverse attack of the hyperactive liver qi or by failure of the stagnated liver qi to perform its dispersing and discharging effect. As a result of upward adverse flow of the gallbladder fire following the rise of the liver fire transformed from the stagnated liver qi, bitter taste in the mouth, intense thirst and vomiting sour or bitter fluid are exhibited.

Therapeutic method: Suppressing the liver to regulate the function of the stomach, and inducing qi to flow downwards to relieve vomiting.

Prescription: Suye Huangliang Tang(Decoction of Perilla and Coptis, from *Compendium on Epidemic Febrile Disease*) with modifications.

Huang Lian(Rhizoma Coptidis) 10g, Wu Mei(Fructus Mume) 10g, Chen Pi(Pericarpium Citri Reticulatae) 9g, Ban Xia(Rhizoma

138

Pinelliae) 9g, Su Ye (Folium Perillae) 9g, Sha Ren (Fructus Amomi) 9g, Mu Xiang (Radix Aucklandiae) 9g, Zhu Ye (Lophatherum) 12g, Fu Ling (Poria) 12g, Ge Gen (Radix Puerariae) 15g, Huan Fen (Radix Trichosanthis) 30g, Gan Cao (Radix Glycyrrhizae) 6g, to be decocted in water for oral dose.

As alternative prescription, Tiaowei Shengjin Zhiou Tang (Decoction for Regulating the Stomach to Generating Body Fluid and Stopping Vomiting, a proved formula developed by Ningbo TCM Hospital) can also be adopted. The ingredients of the formula are:

Zi Su Geng (Caulis Perillae) 10g, Mai Dong (Radix Ophiopogonis) 10g, Wu Mei (Fructus Mume) 2 pieces, Huang Lian (Rhizoma Coptidis) 3g, Zhu Ru (Caulis Bambusae in Taeniam) 6g, Xuan Shen (Radix Scrophulariae) 18g, and Chao Huang Qin (Stir-fried Radix Scutellariae) 5g.

This formula is indicative for morning sickness due to liver heat.

Modifications:

① In case of severe vomiting impairing body fluid marked by red tongue and dry mouth, add Sha Shen (Radix Adenophorae Strictae) 15g, Shi Hu (Herba Dendrobii) 15g and Yu Zhu (Rhizoma Polygonati Odorati) (12g, to nourish the stomach yin.

② If the patient has severe deficiency of both qi and yin, marked by continuous hyperemesis, fever, thirst, oliguria, orbital depression, dull eyes, dryness of lips and tongue, red tongue with dry coating or without coating, rapid, thready and slippery pulse (test of ketone in urine is positive), the treatment should be aimed at supplementing qi and nourishing yin to regulate the function of the stomach and arrest vomiting with the following drugs:

Tai Zi Shen (Radix Pseudostellariae) 30g, Mai Dong (Radix Ophiopogonis Strictae) 15g, Sheng Di (Radix Rehmanniae) 15g, Xuan Shen (Radix Scrophulariae) 15g, Wu Wei Zi (Fructus Schisandrae) 9g, Chen Pi (Pericarpium Citri Reticulatae) 9g, Zhu Ru (Caulis Bambusae in Taeniam) 12g, Tian Hua Fen (Radix Trichosanthis)

30g, Huang Lian (Rhizoma Coptidis) 10g, Huang Qin(Radix Scutellariae) 10g, Sheng Shi Gao (Gypsum Fibrosum) 20g, Gan Cao (Radix Glycyrrhizae) 6g.

The above drugs are to be decocted in water to be taken frequently in small dose by oral use. If a patient has had diabetes before pregancy,oral antihyperlycemic should be stopped and insuline therapy may be implemented instead to correct dehydration, ketoacidosis and electrolyte disorder.

6. 2 Recuperation after delivery

Recuperation must be carried out for those having undergone artificial abortion, habitual abortion,inevitable abortion and normal delivery. Recuperation and nursing should be given respectively according to patient's conditions. As patients used to have general deficiency after delivery, especially deficiency of both qi and blood, unstable blood sugar is usually the main manifestation of gravidic diabetes after delivery.

Main manifestations: Lassitude, shortness of breath, disinclination to talk, lower voice, continuous sweating,aversion to wind, pale and thin tongue coating, feeble and weak pulse, after labour. The blood test shows unstable blood sugar.

Therapeutic method: Supplementing qi, nourishing blood and consolidating the superficies to arrest sweating.

Prescription: Huang Qi(Radix Astragali seu Hedysari) 30g, Bai Zhu (Rhizoma Atractylodis Macrocephalae) 12g, Dang Gui(Radix Angelicae Sinensis) 12g, Dang Shen(Radix Codonopsis Pilosulae) 15g, Fu Ling (Poria) 15g, Fang Feng(Radix Ledebouriellae) 9g, Shu Di(Rhizoma Rehmanniae Praeparatae) 9g, Wu Wei Zi(Fructus Schisandrae) 15g, Shan Yao(Rhizoma Dioscoreae) 15g, Shan Yu Rou(Fructus Cornii) 15g, Hang Shao(Chinese Herbaceous Peony) 15g, Mai Dong (Radix Ophiopogonis) 12g, Gan Cao (Radix Glycyrrhizae) 6g, and Da Zao(Fructus Ziziphi Jujubae) 5 pieces.

The above drugs are to be decocted in water for oral administration.

If the patient has been given oral antihyperglycemia, the dosage should be properly reduced according to the status of blood sugar and the urine sugar. For those having been receiving insulin injection, the dosage needs to be regulated properly according to the status of the blood sugar to prevent hypoglycemia. Breast feeding should be stopped if the diabetes is not well controlled.

Modifications:

① For cases with night sweat, flushed face, red tongue with little coating, which indicates severe consumption of yin and the ensuing generation of interior heat after labour, the treatment should be aimed at nourishing yin, supplementing qi, promoting the generation of body fluid to arrest sweating. The following drugs should be applied:

Ren Shen(Radix Ginseng) 9g, Wu Wei Zi(Fructus Schisandrae) 9g, Mai Dong(Radix Ophiopogonis) 12g, Dang Gui(Radix Angelicae Sinensis) 12g, Fu Xiao Mai(Fructus Tritici Levis) 30g, Mu Li (Concha Ostreae) 30g, and Gan Cao (Radix Glycyrrhizae) 6g, which are to be decocted in water for oral use.

② For cases with postpartum pantalgia due to blood deficiency, the treatment should be aimed at nourishing blood and invigorating qi. The following drugs can be prescribed:

Huang Qi(Radix Astragali seu Hedysari) 30g, Gui Zhi(Ramulus Cinnamomi) 9g, Bai Shao (Radix Paeoniae Alba) 15g, Qin Jiao (Radix Gentianae Macrophyllae) 12g, Dang Gui(Radix Angelicae Sinensis) 12g, Ji Xue Teng(Caulis Spatholobi) 30g, Da Zao(Fructus Ziziphi Jujubae) 5 pieces, and Sheng Jiang(Rhizoma Zingiberis Recens) 3 pieces, to be decocted in water for oral dose.

6.3 Case Study

Li is a 28 year-old female who paid her first visit to our hospital on Oct. 8th, 1989. She compained of two months pregnancy accompanied with anorexia, vomiting, dizziness, and dysphoria, which recently developed into vomiting right after eating, lassitude of the limbs, general weakness with desire for sleep. She was found to have positive ketone in the urine and coffee-like mucus in the vomitus, The above conditions were not relieved by such treatments as fluid transfusion, then she came to seek medical care in our hospital.

Examination showed that she walked under the support of others, and had listlessness, emaciation, disinclination to talk, and constipation for more than half a year, accompanied with feverish sensation, thirst, scanty and dark urine, red and dry tongue with thin and yellowish coating, and thready rapid pulse. Laboratory tests showed that the urine ketone was $++$, the urine sugar $+++$, blood sugar 6. 5mmol/L, and blood pressure, 18/10kPa. Her mother and aunt had a history of diabetes.

TCM diagnosis: Incoordination of the liver and the stomach, gallbladder heat and abnormal discharge of fluid, blood-dryness injuring vessels, and deficieny of both qi and yin-fluid.

Therapeutic method: Regulating the liver and benefiting qi, promoting the production of body fluid to arrest vomiting.

Prescription: Chai Hu (Radix Bupleuri) 6g, Chao Huang Qin (fried Radix Scutellariae) 6g, Huang Lian (Rhizoma Coptidis) 6g, Zi Su Geng (Caulis Perillae) 15g, Gua Lou Pi (Perocarpium Trichosanthis) 15g, Wu Zhu Yu (Fructus Euodiae) 6g, Dang Shen (Radix Codonopsis Pilosulae) 15g, Xuan Shen (Radix Scrophulariae) 18g, Zhu Ru (Caulis Bambusae in Taeniam) 6g, Ban Xia (Rhizoma Pinelliae) 6g, to be decocted in water for immediate use to avoid the further development of the disease.

After two doses administered, she had once bowel movement and the times of vomiting was reduced. She had a better spirit and the amount of urine was increased. But she still had dizziness, nausea with a desire for vomiting, red tongue with thin coating, thready, wiry, slippery but forceless pulse. The urine sugar was detected to be ++, and the ketone in the urine became negative. So the above treatment was continued with the same prescription with modifications:

Dang Shen (Radix Codonopsis Pilosulae) 15g, Xuan Shen (Radix Scrophulariae) 15g, Sheng Di (Radix Rehmanniae) 12g, Mai Dong (Radix Ophiopogonis) 10g, Fu Ling (Poria) 10g, Zi Su Geng (Caulis Perilliae) 10g, Huang Lian (Rhizoma Coptidis) 6g, Zhu Ru (Caulis Bambusae in Taeniam) 9g, Gan Cao (Radix Glycyrrhizae) 3g, Chao Huang Qin (fried Radix Scutellariae) 6g, and Sang Ji Sheng (Ramulus Loranthi) 12g.

After 3 doses administered, she had free bowel movement and vomiting occurred only occasionally. She still had nausea in the morning, and the urine sugar was tested only +. Her blood sugar was not tested. These showed that the condition of the patient had been remarkedly alleviated. To fortify the therapeutic effect, she was instructed to take Xiangsha Liujunzi Wan (Bolus Containing Six Noble Drugs) for three days with the aim of strengthening the spleen qi, and regulating the stomach to prevent abortion. She was also advised to check the blood sugar regularly to observe the changes of her diabetes.

Chapter 7　Common Clinical
Complications of Diabetes

7.1 Diabetic Nephrosis

Diabetic nephrosis is a severe complication of diabetes, which occurs in about $40-50\%$ of the cases with insulin-dependent diabetes and $5-10\%$ of those with non-insulin-dependent diabetes. In recent years, with the prolonging of patients' survival time, diabetic nephrosis occurs more frequently and is being highly evaluated. There is significant difference in the incidence of the complication in the people with different ages and different patterns. About half of the cases with juvenile type died of renal failure, while only about $6-9\%$ of the cases with adult diabetes died of the complication. The cases with non-insulin-dependent diabetes died from the complication are even less. They mostly died from the complication of the cardiovascular diseases, and even if they have nephrosis, they also have primary hypertension and atherosclerosis.

The complications of the diabetes may involve every system and viscera. It is directly related to the vascular disorders caused by diabetes. According to statistics in China, 90% of the renal biopsy on patients with diabetes showed positive results. Therefore, diabetic nephrosis has become an important subject of modern medical science.

The mechanism of the disease is still unclear and there is not specific treatment in Western medicine at present. However, application of the herbal medicines to promote blood flow and remove blood stasis and promote the discharge of turbid substance from the fu organs may reverse, delay and terminate the development of the disease

144

while the diabetes and hypertension are effectively controlled.

Although there is no direct record of the disease in the ancient liter-ature, the complications of Xiaoke (Diabetes) such as edema and blurred vision had been long treated and recognized. *Sheng Ji Zong Lu* (General Collection for Holy Relief) states: "The kidney impairment in diabetes patients will cause disturbance of the transforming effect of the kidney as a result of the kidney qi deficiency. Consequently, the kidney fails to control the opening and closing of the bladder and water retains to lead to edema", and "Diabetes is likely to change. If it is not cured for a long time, edema may be caused."

According to TCM, the diabetic nephrosis is caused by kidney qi de-ficiency and blood stasis due to the lingering course of the diabetes. Its pathogenesis is characterized by disorders of the liver and the kidney due to yin deficiency in the initial stage, deficiency of both the spleen yang and the kidney yang later due to yin deficiency affecting yang, which leads to retention of water and its overflow to the skin and mus-cles, and deficiency of the kidney yang in the later stage which caus-es overflow of water, stagnation of turbid toxic substances and their upward attack on the heart and the lung. In the later stage, there are dyspnea, inability to lie flat, or even depletion of both yin and yang or exhaustion of yang as a consequence of yin consumption. In the whole course of the disease, qi deficiency and blood stasis occupy an important role, and apart from the liver, the spleen and the kidney, the heart, the lung and the triple-jiao are also involved.

7. 1. 1 Deficiency of the liver yin and the kidney yin complicated by blood stasis

Main manifestations: Lassitude, feverish sensation over the soles, palms and chest, dry mouth and throat, dry eyes, blurred vision, soreness of the loins and knees, dizziness, tinnitus, mild edema of the face and feet, frequent and profuse urine, dark red lips and tongue, wiry rapid pulse, positive urinary protein and small amount of exu-date on optical fundus.

145

Therapeutic method: Nourishing the liver and the kidney, promoting blood flow and removing blood stasis.

Prescription: Qiju Dihuang Tang (Bolus of Fructus Lycii, Flos Crysanthemi and Rhizoma Rehmanniae Praeparatae) with modification.

Gou Qi (fructus Lycii) 12g, Shu Di (Rhizoma Rehmanniae Praeparatae) 12g, Shan Yao (Rhizoma Dioscoreae) 12g, Mai Dong (Radix Ophiopogonis) 12g, Shan Yu Rou (Fructus Cornii) 12g, Ju Hua (Flos Crysanthemi) 9g, Dang Gui (Radix Angelcae Sinensis) 15g, Chi Shao (Radix Paeoniae Rubra) 15g, Yi Mu Cao (Herba Leonuri) 30g, Dan Shen (Radix Salviae Miltiorrhizae), Tai Zi Shen (Radix Pseudostellariae) 30g, Ze Xie (Rhizoma Alismatis) 30g, Ze Lan (Herba Lycopi) 30g, Da Huang (Radix et Rhizoma Rhei) 6g, to be decocted in water for oral dose.

The treatment may be modified based on the prescription and should continue for more than six months. Besides, small dose of insulin and Diamicron can be administered to control the blood sugar. During the administration, changes of blood pressure must be noticed.

Modifications in accordance with symptoms:

① In the cases of overabundant heat in the stomach and the lung after the treatment, marked by dry mouth, thirst, or polyphagia and polydipsia, add Hua Fen (Radix Trichosanthis) 30g, Yuan Shen (Radix Scrophulariae) 15g and Ge Gen (Radix Pueriae) 20g.

② For cases with obvious qi deficiency, add Huang Qi (Radix Astragali seu Hedysari) 30g and Wu Wei Zi (Fructus Schisanthis) 10g to supplement qi and nourish yin so that vigorous qi can promote flow of blood.

③ In the cases of no alleviation of edema with increased urine protein, add Dong Gua Pi (Exocarpium Benincasae) 30g, Chi Xiao Dou (Semen Phaseoli) 15g, Niu Xi (Radix Achyranthis) 15g, and Jin Ying Zi (Fructus Rosae Laevigatae) 15g.

④ For those with severe yin deficiency, add Gui Ban Jiao (Colla

146

Plastri Testudinis) 15g, Niu Zhen Zi(Fructus Ligustici Lucidi) 20g and Han Lian Ye(Herba Ecliptae) 12g.

⑤ For those with loose stool, add Can Zhu(Rhizoma Atractylodis) 15g and Lian Zi Rou(Semen Nelumbinis) 20g. For protracted diarrhea, Shen Ling Bai Zhu San(Powder of Radix Ginseng, Poria and Rhizoma Atractylodis Macrocephalae, from *Prescriptions of Peaceful Benevolent Dispensary*) or Si Shen Wan(Four Miraculous Drugs Bolus, from *Standards of Diagnosis and Treatment*) can be taken in combination.

⑥ For those with hypertension, marked by severe dizziness, add Tian Ma(Rhizoma Gastrodiae) 15g and Gou Teng(Ramulus Uncariae cum Uncis) 18g, or administer the hypotensor.

⑦ For those with severe retinal lesion marked by blurring of vision, add Shi Hu(Herba Dendrobii) 12g, Shi Jue Ming(Concha Haliotidis) 30g and Gu Jing Cao(Flos Eriocauli) 15g.

⑧ If urinary stone or infection is detected, active treatment should be taken to prevent the further development of the condition.

7. 1. 2 Deficiency of both the spleen yang and the kidney yang accompanied with blood stasis

Main manifestations : Lassitude, soreness and pain of the loins and knees, edema of the face and feet, aversion to cold and cold limbs, blurred vision, loose stool, palpiatation, spontaneous sweating, poor appetite, nausea, abdominal distension, frequent urine at night, dark, tender and enlarged tongue with teeth print and thready feeble pulse.

Patients in this stage usually have a high blood sugar, reduced urine glucose, obviously increased proteinuria, oliguria, and obvious hypopsia. Besides, they may have complications such as hypertension, atherosclerosis, manifested as bleeding, increased whitish exudates and ceroid form of veins on the optical fundus.

Therapeutic method : Replenishing both the spleen and the kidney, warming up yang to induce diuresis, assisted by promoting blood flow and removing blood stasis.

Prescription: Huang Qi(Radix Astragali seu Hedysari) 30g, Dang Shen (Radix Codonopsis Pilosulae) 20g, Shan Yao (Rhizoma Dioscoreae) 20g, Zhu Ling(Polyporus Umbellatus) 30g, Fu Ling Pi (Poria Peel) 30g, Ze Xie (Rhizoma Alismatis) 30g, Ze Lan(Herba Lycopi) 30g, Dan Shen (Radix Salviae Miltiorrhizae) 30g, Xian Ling Pi(Herba Epimedii) 15g, Shan Yu Rou(Fructus Cornii) 15g, Mu Gua(Fructus Chaenomelis) 15g, Gui Zhi(Ramulus Cinamomi) 6g, Fu Zi (Radix Aconiti Praeparata) 10g, and Hong Hua (Flos Carthami) 10g, to be decocted in water for oral use.

This recipe can be long administered with proper modifications. If the blood sugar and the blood pressure is well controlled, the recipe can relieve the disease condition or prevent it from deterioration.

Modifications in accordance with symptoms:

①In the case with impairment of both qi and yin, the recipe can be substituted for: Shu Di (Radix Rehmanniae Praeparatae) 15g, Shan Yao(Rhizoma Dioscoreae) 15g, Huang Jing(Rhizoma Polygonati) 15g, Ze Xie(Rhizoma Alismatis) 15g, Shan Yu Rou(Fructus Cornii) 15g, Dan Pi (Cortex Moutan Radicis) 9g, Dang Shen (Radix Codonopsis Pilosulae) 20g and Huang Qi(Radix Astragali seu Hedysari) 30g, to be decocted in water for oral dose.

② For those with deficiency of the kidney essence, the treatment should be directed at nourishing the kidney yin by the support of strengthening the spleen to eliminate dampness and removing blood stasis in the collaterals. Liu Wei Di Huang Tang (Decoction of Six Drugs Containing Radix Rehmanniae, from *Key to Therapeutics of Children's Disease*) plus Huang Jing(Rhizoma Polygonati) 15g, Ji Xue Teng(Caulis Spatholobi) 15g, Cang Zhu(Rhizoma Atractylodis) 20g and Yi Yi Ren(Semen Coicis) 15g can be administered.

③ For those with deiciency of both the spleen and kidney marked by diarrhea, the treatment should be aimed at strengthening the spleen to induce diuresis, remvoing blood stasis and benifiting the kidney. The commonly used drugs are:

Dang Shen(Radix Codonopsis Pilosulae) 15g, Shan Yao(Rhizoma Dioscoreae) 15g, Fu Ling(Poria) 15g, Jiao Bai Zhu(Parched Rhizoma Atractylodis Macrocephalae) 15g, Chao Ge Gen (Stir-fried Radix Puerariae) 15g, Chao Bian Dou(Stir-fried Semen Dolicaris) 30g, Chao Chen Pi(Stir-fried Pericarpium Citri Reticulatae), Chao Che Qian Zi (Stir-fried Semen Plantaginis) 30g, and Mi Ke(Rice Bran) 9g,to be decocted in water for oral dose. After recovery from diarrhea, the patient should be given the original recipe to treat diabetes.

④ If the condition is manifested as deficiency of the spleen qi and the kidney qi, the treatment should be to strengthen the spleen and consolidate the kidney with Shui Lu Er Xian Dan(Bolus Both Inducing Diuresis and Loosing the Bowel), which is composed of Jin Ying Zi(Fructus Rosae Laevigatae) 30g and Qian Shi(Semen Euryales) 15g, Qianshi Mixture, which consists of Qian Shi (Semen Eurygalis), Bai Zhu (Rhizoma Atractylodis Macrocephalae), Fu Ling (Poria), Shan Yao (Rhizoma Dioscoreae), Huang Jing (Rhizoma Poligonati), Tu Si Zi(Semen Cuscutae), Jin Ying Zi(Fructus Rosae Laevigatae), Bai He(Bulbus Lilii), and Pi Pa Ye(Folium Eribotryae), or Bu Zhong Yi Qi Tang (Decoction of Strengthening Middle-Jiao and Benefiting Qi, from *Treatise on the Spleen and Stomach*) with Jin Ying Zi(Fructus Rosae Laevigatae) 15g,Bu Gu Zhi(Fructus Psoraleae) 15g and Tu Si Zi(Semen Cuscutae) 15g added.

⑤ For those with severe edema, add Niu Xi(Radix Achyranthis Bidentatae) 30g, Che Qian Zi(Semen Plantaginis) 30g, Chi Xiao Dou (Semen Phasaoli) 30g, Dong Gua Pi(Exocarpium Benincasae) 30g, and Fang Ji(Radix Stephaniae Tetrandrae) 12g. Ji Sheng Shen Qi Wan (Benevolent Pills for Supplementing Kidney Qi, from *Prescriptions for Benovalence*) can also be adopted as an alternative.

7. 1. 3 Deficiency of the five zang organs and accumulation of turbid toxin in the interior

149

Main manifestations: On the basis of the manifestations of deficiency of both the spleen Yang and the kidney yang, edema becomes more and more severe and is accompanied with aversion to cold, cold limbs, oliguria, pale complexion, asthma with inability to lie flat, epigastric and abdominal fullness, loss of appetite, vomiting, nausea, and deep and weak pulse.

This type is caused by deficiency of the five zang organs and the ensuing dysfunction of the spleen and inability of the kidney to warm and steam water. As a result, water fails to be distributed freely and accumulates in the body, giving rise to stagnation and interlocking of turbid dampness in triple-jiao. In this case, the turbid dampness attacks the heart and the lung in the upper, influences the ascending-descending movement of qi of the spleen and stomach and leads to failure of the turbid to be separated from the clear in the middle, and obstruction of the pathway of urine and the resultant internal accumulation of turbid toxin in the lower. As the turbid toxin is unable to be discharged, the condition is rather severe.

Therapeutic method: Benefiting qi, tonifying the kidney, nourishing yin and supporting yang, activating blood flow and removing blood stasis, eliminating the turbid by loosing the bowl.

Prescription: Huang Qi(Radix Astragali) 30g, Ze Lan(Herba Lycopi) 30g, Sheng Di (Radix Rehmanniae) 12g, Shu Di (Radix Rehmanniae Praeparatae) 12g, Xian Ling Pi(Herba Epimedii) 12g, Xian Mao(Rhizoma Curculiginis) 12g, Shan Yao(Rhizoma Dioscoreae) 15g, Dang Gui(Radix Angelicae Sinensis) 15g, Chi Shao(Radix Paeoniae Rubra) 15g, Hong Hua (Flos Carthami) 15g, Dan Shen (Radix Salviae Miltiorrhizae) 30g, Ge Gen (Radix Puaeriariae) 20g, Da Huang(Radix et Rhizoma Rhei) 9g(to be decocted later), to be decocted in water for roal dose.

Modifications in accordance with symtoms:

① For cases with retained water-dampness attacking the heart and the lung, the treatment should be aimed at warming up the kidney and strengthening the heart to promote distribution of water, activating blood flow and removing blood stasis, and lowering the turbid and dissolving phlegm. The following herbs should be prescribed:

Fu Ling (Poria) 30g, Bai Zhu (Rhizoma Atractylodis Macrocephalae)15g, Ting Ling Zi (Semen Lepidii seu Descurainiae) 15g, Dan Shen (Radix Salviae Miltiorrhizae) 15g, Chao Zao Ren (Stir-fried Semen Ziziphi Spinosae) 15g, Ze Lan (Herba Lycopi) 30g, Gui Zhi (Ramulus Cinnamomi) 10g, Sang Bai Pi (Cortex Mori Radicis) 12g, and Gan Cao (Radix Glycyrrhizae) 6g, to be decocted in water for oral dose.

② For cases with stagnation of the liver qi, marked by bitter taste in the mouth and hypochondriac pain, add Chai Hu (Radix Bupleuri) 12g, Zhi Ke (Fructus Aurantii) 10g, and Yu Jin (Radix Curcumae) 12g.

③ For cases with erythrocyte and leukocyte in the urine and urgent, frequent and painful urination, add Bai Mao Gen (Rhizoma Imperatae) 30g, Shi Wei (Folium Pyrrosiae) 30g, Che Qian Zi (Semen Plantaginis, packed) 30g, Di Yu (Radix Sanguisorbae) 15g, Dong Kui Zi (Fructus Malvae Vertillatae) 15g, Xiao Ji (Herba Cephalanoploris) 15g, Kun Cao (Herba Lonnuri) 15g, Hua Shi (Talcum) 15g, and Pi Xie (Rhizoma Dioscoreae Hypoglaucae) 12g.

④ For cases with urinaemia, manifested as nausea, vomiting, and yellow thick tongue coating, the original recipe should be substituted for Huang Lian Wen Dan Tang (Rhizoma Coptidis Decoction for Warming Gallbladder) with modification, which includes: Huang Lian (Rhizoma Coptidis) 10g, Jiang Ban Xia (Rhizoma Pinelliae, prepared with ginger) 10g, Chen Pi (Pericarpium Citri Reticulatae) 10g, Zhi Shi (Fructus Aurantii Immaturus) 10g, Su Geng (Caulis Perillae) 10g, Fu Ling (Poria) 15g, Zhu Ru (Caulis Bambusae in Taeniam) 12g, Gan Cao (Radix Glycyrrhizae) 6g, and Sheng Jiang (Rhizoma Zingiberis Recens) 3 pieces, to be decocted in water for oral dose.

151

⑤ For cases with gingival bleeding and epistaxis, add Bai Mao Gen(Rhizoma Imperatae) 30g, Ou Jie(Nodus Nelumbinis Rhizomalis) 30g, Sheng Di Tang(Radix Rehmanniae, carbonized) 15g, Xiao Ji(Herba Cephalanoploris) 15g, and Dan Pi (Cortex Moutan Radicis) 12g.

This type refers to advanced diabetic nephrosis or renal failure with turbid toxin accumulating in the interior. According to TCM, it is a syndrome deficiency in origin and excess in superficiality and deficiency complicated by excess. The deficiency in origin here indicates deficiency of both yin and yang of the kidney and the deficiency of other organs, while the excess in superficiality, the obstruction of coagulated blood in the collaterals and accumulation of turbid toxin in the interior. This two aspects have a causative- resultant relationship, which eventually leads to weakness of all the five zang organs and exhaustion of yin and yang. For this type, the treatment should be aimed at supporting the vital qi and eliminating pathogenic factors or treating both the origin and superficiality. The commonly used drugs include: Huang Qi(Radix Astragali), Ren Shen(Radix Ginseng.), Bai Zhu (Rhizoma Atractylodis Macrocephalae), Zhu Ling(Polyporus), Fu Ling(Poria), Ze Xie(Rhizoma Alismatis), Shan Yao(Rhizoma Dioscoreae), Xian Ling Pi(Herba Epimedii), Shu Fu Zi(Radix Aconiti Praeparatae), Xian Mao(Rhizoma Curculiginis), Sheng Di(Radix Rehmanniae), Gou Qi(Fructus Lycii), Shan Yu Rou(Fructus Cornii), Wu Wei Zi(Fructus Schisandrae), Dang Gui(Radix Angelicae Sinensis), Dan Shen (Radix Salviae Miltiorrhizae), Chi Shao(Radix Paeoniae Rubra), Kun Cao(Herba Lonnuri), Chi Xiao Dou(Semen Phaseoli), Yu Mi Xu(Semen Maydis), Qian Shi(Semen Euryales), Shi Wei(Folium Pyrrosiae), Che Qian Zi(Semen Plantaginis), etc. , which can be adopted deliberately.

At present, there is still no special therapy for diabetic nephrosis, because its cause is not clear enough. Western medicine aims the treatment at the control of symptoms, or the control of the blood sugar, the blood pressure, and the blood viscosity and the prevention and treatment of the vascular lesions. But such treatments could not reverse the disease development. In some severe cases, dialysis and kidney transplantation may be an effective therapy, but as they cost much money, they could not be widely applied and could work not as a preventive treatment as well. Therefore, TCM therapy should be adopted on the basis of syndrome identification. At the early stage, the key to the prevention of the occurrence and development of diabetic nephrosis lies in the the treatment of primary disease, control of the blood sugar, blood lipid and blood pressure, regulation of the metabolism of sugar, fat, and protein, as well as the treatment of various kinds of urinary infections and prostatic diseases. At the later stage in which the diseases becomes rather complicated and extremely severe, combined Chinese and Western medicine should be employed to treat the fetal complications such as uriremia and heart failure.

7. 1. 4 Case Study

Chen is a 60 years old male worker of a factory in Lin Qu county who was admitted in July, 1985, complaining of polyphagia, polydipsia and polyuria for fifteen years which were aggravated in the previous half a year. His registered number was 85106, and the admission diagnosis was diabetes.

When he was hospitalized, his fasting blood sugar was 13. 66mmol/L. Through proper treatment, polyphagia, polydipsia and polyuria were gradually alleviated. But on Sept. 7th, 1988, he experienced sudden dizziness, headache and vomiting, followed by listlessness, apathy, divagation, edema of the legs, dark and tender tongue with whitish glossy coating, and deep thready pulse. Laboratory test revealed that BUN was 2. 28 mmol/ L, and the urine protein +++. Then he was diagnosed as having diabetic nephrosis complicated by chronic urinaemia. Correspondingly, he was treated with combined Chinese and Western medicine to support his life, induce diuresis, and promote discharge of toxic materials by loosing the bowel

153

for more than two months. But the condition was not controlled and had developed further. BUN raised to be 37. 35mmol/L and the serum potassium, 5. 5mmol/L. Considering that the main pathological changes of diabetic nephrosis was glomerular atherioscelerosis according to Western medicine and phlegm was responsible for a great many of diseases according to TCM, drugs softening hardness to dissipate masses and activateing blood flow to remove blood stasis were given. The recipe prescribed consisted of:

Kun Bu(Thallus Laminariae) 20g, Hai Zao(Sargassum) 15g, Xuan Shen (Radix Scrophulariae) 12g, Sheng Jiang (Rhizoma Zingiberis Recens) 20g, Zhe Bei(Bulbus Fritillariae Thunbergii) 30g, Sheng Mu Li(Concha Ostreae) 30g, Fu Ling(Poria) 30g, Kun Cao (Herba Lonnuri) 6g and Tao Ren (Semen Persicae) 15g, to be decocted in water for frequent use in small doses. After 10 doses were administered, headache, dizziness and vomiting disappeared. After 20 more doses were administered, his spirit and consciousness restored to normal, urine increased and edema relieved. Reexamination showed that UBN decreased to 21. 4mmol/L, electrolyte was normal, amd protein in the urine disappeared. Then he was continuously treated with the purpose to fortify the therapeutic effect for three months before his discharge. (From *Experience in Treating Intractable Diabetes*, written by Wei Shoukuan, et)

Notes: The main pathological basis of diabetic nephrosis is the glomerular atherosclerosis, which is considered a unreversible pathological change very difficult to treat in Western medicine. Even such Western therapy as renal dialysis and the TCM therapy as promoting discharge of the turbid by loosing the bowel cannot be effective. However, unexpected effect had been obtained in the treatment of this case based on a diagnosis of both disease and syndrome by softening hardness and removing blood stasis, which is a success of the combined use of both Chinese and Western medicine. This opened a new road which is worth further researching for the treatment of the disease. (From *Experience in Treating Intractable Diabetes*, by Wei Shoukuan, et. al)

7. 2 Diabetes and hypertension

The incidence of hypertention among diabetes patients is much higher than that among others, which is common in any parts of the world. It is reported from abroad that the incidence reaches $40-50\%$ of the diabetes patients. According to the reports from China, it is four times that of the other populations in Shanghai and 5 times that of the other populations in Beijing. The disease is rather complicated and its mechanism is still unknown. Diabetic patients complicated by hypertension have a tendency to suffer from cerebrovascular accidents, coronary heart disease and hypertensive heart disease. And diabetes, especially that complicated by hypertension, often serves as the most important cause of cerebrovascular accident. By now there is still no radical therapy for the disease, the oral hypertensors can only control the blood pressure in a lower range but cannot cure it. However, effective prevention and treatment of diabetes and hypertension will be beneficial to the prvention of the early renal lesions and the diseases of the optical fundus, and can help to postpone the occurrence of renal failure and asthenopia. As a fundamental measure, treating diabetes must be stressed apart from the treatment of hypertension. According to TCM, the pathogenesis of hypertension in diabetes consists in deficiency of zang-fu organs, imbalance between yin and yang or accumulation of phlegm-turbid in the middle-jiao, which result from emotional stress or sudden rage, improper diet, overfeeding or underdue feeding, over fatigue or constitution variation, and the subsequent deficiency of vital qi. Therefore, the fundamental of the disease is deficiency of the vital qi. The commonly seen types include hyperactivity of the liver yang, deficiency of both the liver yin and the kidney yin, and accumulation of phlegm-turbid in the interior. And the treatment should be mainly aimed at reinforcing the deficien-

155

cy and reducing the excess. Besides, diabetes must be treated properly.

Syndrome identification and corresponding treatment are as following:

7.2.1 Hyperactivity of the liver yang

Main manifestations: Dizziness, tinnitus, headache, distension of the head, flushing of face, irritability, insomnia, dream-disturbed sleep, bitter taste in the mouth and dry throat, red tongue with yellow coating, rapid and wiry pulse, increased blood sugar.

Therapeutic method: Suppressing the hyperactive yang and nourishing the liver and the kidney.

Prescription: Tian Ma (Rhizoma Castrodiae, to be decocted first) 15g, Gou Teng (Ramulus Uncariae cum Uncis, to be decocted later) 18g, Sheng Shi Jue Ming (Concha Haliotidis) 30g, Ye Jiao Teng (Caulis Polygoni Multiflori) 30g, Chao Zao Ren (Stir-fried Fructus Ziziphi Spinosae) 30g, Huang Qin (Radix Scutellariae) 12g, Zhi Zi (Fructus Gardeniae) 9g, Du Zhong (Cortex Eucommiae) 9g, Niu Xi (Radix Achyranthis Bidentatae) 15g, Fu Sheng (Poria cum Ligno Hospite) 15g, Yi Mu Cao (Herba Leonuri) 15g, and Sang Ji Sheng (Ramulus Loranthi) 20g, to be decocted in water for oral dose.

Modifications in accordance with symptoms:

① For cases marked by polydipsia, add Hua Fen (Radix Trichosanthis) 30g and Zhi Mu (Rhizoma Anemarrhenae) 15g.

② For cases marked by polyphagia, add Huang Lian (Rhizoma Coptidis) 10g and Cang Zhu (Rhizoma Atractylodis) 20g.

③ For cases with severe yin deficiency, add Sheng Di (Radix Rehmanniae) 15g, Mai Dong (Radix Ophiopogonis) 15g, Xuan Shen (Radix Scrophulariae) 15g, Shou Wu (Radix Polygoni Multiflori) 15g and Sheng Bai Shao (Radix Paeoniae Alba) 15g deliberately.

④ For cases with numbness or even tremor of limbs, add Zhen Zhu Mu (Concha Margarilifera Usta) or Ling Yang Jiao Fen (Cornu

156

Antelopis), etc.

⑤ In the case of generation of endogenous wind due to fire, or stirring of the liver wind, apoplexia may appear. The mild cases are marked by numbness of the limbs, tremor of the limbs, and distortion of eyes and mouth; while the severe cases, by sudden coma, unconsciousness, aphasia, and hemiplegia. For such cases, the recipe should be substituted for Ling Yang Gou Teng Tang (Decoction of Cornu Antelopis and Ramulus Uncariae cum Uncis) with Quan Xie (Scorpio), Di Long (Lumbricus), Wu Gong (Scolopendra), or Jiang Can (Bombyx Batryticatus) added to suppress the liver wind and relieve convulsion.

7. 2. 2 Deficiency of both the liver yin and the kidney yin

Main manifestations: Dizziness, vertigo, blurring of vision, soreness of the loins and knees, insomnia, dream-disturbed sleep, palpitation, dysphoria, forgetfulness, red tongue with little coating, and wiry thready pulse.

Therapeutic method: Nourishing the liver and the kidney.

Prescription: Gou Qi (Fructus Lycii) 12g, Ju Hua (Flos Chrysanthemi) 10g, Sheng Di (Radix Rehmanniae) 15g, Shan Yao (Rhizoma Dioscoreae) 15g, Shan Yu Rou (Fructus Corni) 15g, Fu Ling (Poria) 15g, Ze Xie (Rhizoma Alismatis) 15g, Hang Shao (Chinese Herbaceous Peony) 15g, Ge Gen (Radix Pueriariae) 15g, Dan Pi (Cortex Moutan Radicis) 10g, Shou Wu (Radix Polygoni Multiflori) 20g, Sang Ji Sheng (Ramulus Loranthi) 20g, Huai Niu Xi (Radix Achyranthis Bidentatae) 20g, Dan Shen (Radix Salviae Miltiorrhizae) 30g, and Gan Cao (Radix Glycyrrhizae) 6g, to be decocted in water for oral dose.

Modifications in accordance with symptoms:

① For cases marked by kidney yin deficiency, administer Zuo Gui Wan (Pill for Nourishing the Kidney Yin) in the form of decoction to tonify the kidney and supplement the essence.

② In the case of kidney yin deficiency causing heat marked by feverish sensation over the palms, soles and chest, etc. , add Zhi Bie Jia (Stir- fried Carapax Trionycis), Zhi Mu (Rhizoma Anemarrhenae), Huang Bai(Cortex Phellodendri), etc. to Zuo Gui Wan to nourish Yin and clear heat.

③ For cases with hyperactivity of the liver yang due to kidey yin deficiency, the treatment may be performed based on that for hyperactivity of the liver yang with the drugs nourishing the liver and kidney properly added.

④ For cases with incoordination between the heart and the kidney marked by insomnia, dream-disturbed sleep and forgetfulness, add E Jiao(Colla Corii Asini), Ji Zi Huang(Yolk), Suan Zao Ren(Fructus Ziziphi Spinosae), Bai Zi Ren (Semen Biotae), etc. to Zuo Gui Wan to restore the normal coordination between the heart and the kidney.

⑤ For cases with severe dry mouth and thirst, which indicates deficiency of the lung yin, Sha Shen (Radix Adenophorae Strictae), Mai Dong (Radix Ophiopogonis), Yu Zhu (Rhizoma Polygonati Odorati), etc. should be added to nourish the lung yin.

7. 2. 3 Stagnation of phlegm-dampness in the middle jiao

Main manifestations: Dizziness, heaviness of the head as if being bounded, oppressed feeling over the chest, nausea, poor appetite, sleepiness, whitish greasy tongue coating and soft pulse.

Therapeutic method: Drying dampness, eliminating phlegm, strengthening the spleen and regulating the function of the stomach.

Prescription: Ban Xia (Rhizoma Pinelliae) 10g, Chen Pi (Pericarpium Citri Reticulatae) 9g, Fu Ling(Poria) 15g, Bai Zhu(Rhizoma Atrctylodis Macrocephalae) 15g, Tian Ma(Rhizoma Gastrodiae, to be decocted first and then taken with the decoction of the other ingredients), Yi Ren (Semen Coicis) 15g, Man Jing Zi(Fructus Viticis) 10g, Shi Chang Pu (Rhizoma Acori Graminei) 12g, Pei Lan(Herba Eupatorii) 12g, Gan Cao (Radiix Glycyrrhizae) 6g, Sheng Jiang (Rhizoma Zingiberis Recens) 3 pieces, and Da Zao(Fructus Ziziphi

158

Jujubae) 5 pieces, to be decocted in water for oral dose.

Modifications in accordance with symptoms:

① For cases with severe dizziness due to hypertension accompanied with nausea and vomiting, add Dai Zhe Shi (Ochra Haematitum) 15g and Zhu Ru(Caulis Bambusae in Taeniam) 12g to regulate the stomach and lower the upward adverse flow of the stomach qi.

② For cases with discomfort over the epigastriac region and abdominal fullness and distension, add Bai Kou Ren (Semen Amomi Cardamomi) 12g, Sha Ren(Fructus Amomi) 10g and Mu Xiang(Radix Aucklandiae) 10g to regulate the flow of qi and remove dampness.

③ For cases with severe dizziness,tinnitus and poor hearing due to dampness obstructing the upper orifices, add Cong Bai(Bulbus Allii) 3 inches, Yu Jin(Radix Curcumae)12g and Shi Chang Pu(Rhizoma Acori Graminei)12g to activate yang and smooth the orifices.

④ For cases with distending pain of the head, dysphoria, bitter taste in the mouth, dry mouth but not desire for drinking, yellow and greasy tongue and wiry slippery pulse caused by the heat transformed from the phlegm, add Huang Lian (Rhizoma Coptidis) and Zhu Ru(Caulis Bambusae in Taeniam) to dissolve phlegm and clear heat. Modified Huang Lian Wen Dan Tang (Coptis Decoction for Warming the Gallbladder) can also be used as an alternative.

⑤ In the case of the turbid-dampness impairing the spleen yang, marked by abdominal distension, diarrhea and whitish greasy tongue coating, add Gan Jiang(Rhizoma Zingiberis) and Rou Dou Kou(Semen Myristicae) to warm up the spleen yang and arrest diarrhea. Modified Shen Ling Bai Zhu San(Powder of Radix Ginseng, Poria and Rhizoma Atractylodis Macrocephalae)can also be applied.

⑥ For cases with palpitation, and knotted or intermittent pulse due to obstruction of the heart yang by phlegm-dampness, add Shi Chang Pu(Rhizoma Acor Graminei) 12g, Yu Jin(Radix Curcumae) 12g, Suan Zao Ren(Fructus Ziziphi Spinosae) 30g, Zhu Sha Fen

(Powder of Cinnabaris), to be taken with water)and Gui Zhi(Ramulus Cinnamomi)9g to activate yang and dissolve phlegm, tranquilize the mind to arrest mental stress.

⑦ If hemiplegia occurs as a result of the further development of hypertension and diabetes which causes phlegm obstructing in the brain, first aid should be given to treat the hemiplegia first.

7. 2. 4 Case Study

Case 1.

Liu was a 52 year-old female peasant who was diagnosed as diabetes and hypertension in a hospital in June, 1985, where she complaint of polydipsia, polyuria and emaciation. The examinations showd that her fasting blood sugar was 18. 3mmol/L, the urine glucose was +++ and the blood pressure was 27/13kPa. She was treated with glybenzcyclamide, Xiaoke Bolus, Compound Hypotensor, Luobuma, etc. , which decreased the sugar in the urine temporarily (the blood sugar was not rechecked). However, the urine sugar would increase if the drugs were stopped or the amounts were reduced. In the previous two months, she had a subjective feeling of dizziness, headache, dysphoria, palpitation or even tachycardia, irritability, thirst with desire for drinks, dry eyes, dry stool, frequent urination, dark red tongue with little coating, and wiry rapid pulse. Her blood pressure was 24/13kPa. So she was diagnosed as having Xiaoke and dizziness due to depletion of the liver yin and the kidney yin and insufficiency of the heart yin in the light of TCM.

Therapeutic method: Nourishing the kidney and softening the liver, nourishing yin to suppress the hyperactive yang, supported by calming the mind by nourishing the heart.

Prescription:

① Gou Qi(Fructus Lycii) 12g, Shan Yao(Rhizoma Dioscoreae) 12g, Shan Yu Rou(Fructus Corni) 12g, Mai Dong(Radix Ophiopogonis) 12g, Bai Zi Ren (Semen Biotae) 12g, Ju Hua (Flos Chrysanthemi) 9g, Dan Pi(Cortex Moutan Radicis) 9g, Fu Ling(Po-

160

ria） 10g, Ze Xie （Rhizoma Alismatis） 10g, Hua Fen（Radix Tri-
chosanthis） 30g, Chao Zao Ren（Stir-fried Fructus Ziziphi Spinosae）
30g, Sheng Di（Radix Rehmanniae） 15g, Xuan Shen（Radix Scrophu-
lariae） 15g, and Gan Cao（Radix Glycyrrhizae） 6g, to be decocted
for oral use.

② Xiaoke Pills, 10 pills each time, three times daily.

③ Xiaoke Ping, 8 tablets each time, three times daily.

The patient was also advised to stop the Compound Hypotensor temporarily and control her diet, eating only 150 grams of staple food.
After taking the decoction for 15 doses, she made her second visit.
Dry mouth was relieved, the blood pressure decreased to 20/13kPa,
and the fasting blood sugar was reduced from ＋＋＋ to ＋＋ and
further to ＋. She still had bitter taste in the mouth. So Huang Lian
（Rhizoma Coptidis） 10g was added to the recipe. After more fifteen
doses were administered, her fasting blood sugar decreased to
10mmol/L, the fasting urine sugar was ＋ and ＋＋ two hours after
meal, and the blood pressure was reduced to 21/12/kPa. Her other
symptoms were also relieved, palpitation became less severe. She still
had blurring of vision, which was diagnosed as diabetic cataract
through ophthalmological examination. Consequently, she was prescribed Zhangyan Ming, to be taken 4 tablets each time, three times
daily, and Bainei Ting（Drop for Treating Cataracta） for external application. The Chinese herbs were those supplementing qi, tonifying
the kidney, and nourishing yin to clear away heat, which included:

Huang Qi（Radix Astragali seu Hedysari） 30g, Shu Di （Radix
Rehmanniae Praeparatae） 30g, Sha Yu Rou（Fructus Corni） 20g,
Shan Yao （Rhizoma Dioscoreae） 15g, Hang Shao（Chinese Herba-
ceous Peony） 15g, Ge Gen（Radix Pueriariae） 15g, Xuan Shen
（Radix Scrophulariae） 15g, Gou Qi （Fructus Lycii） 12g, Shi Hu
（Herba Dendrobii） 12g, Dan Shen （Radix Salviae Miltiorrhizae）
30g, Hua Fen（Radix Trichosanthis） 30g, Ju Hua （Flos Chrysanthe-
mi） 9g, Huang Lian（Rhizoma Coptidis） 10g and Gan Cao （Radix

Glycyrrhizae) 6g, to be decocted in water for oral dose.

The above treatments was continued for two months or more, her blood was kept around 20/12kPa and repeated examination showed that the blood sugar was $7-8$ mmol/L and the fasting urine glucose (-) . Then the decoction was stopped and Xiaoke Wan(Bolus for Treating Diabetes) which was to be taken 8 tablets each time, three times daily, and Xiaoke Ping(Diabetes Controller) which was to be taken 8 tablets each time, three times daily, and Qi Ju Di Huang Wan (Bolus of Fructus Lycii and Flos Chrysanthemi and Radix Rehmanniae), which was to be taken 1 bolus each time, three times daily, were prescribed to be applied in a longer time. In addition, she was advised to undergo an operation after full development of the phacoscotasmus.

Case 2.

Wang was a 62 year-old female retired official clerk who had been ill with diabetes for 7 years. She compaint of dry mouth, thirst with little drinking, dizziness, vertigo, palpitation, shortness of breath,oppressed feeling in the chest, and paroxysmal cardiac pain radiating to the back. He was diagnosed as having diabetes complicated by hypertension and coronary heart disease in another hostipal, and was given many kinds of Western medicines for reducing blood sugar, hypertension and nitroglycerin, which were not effective. Then,she came to our hospital in Janurary 15,1991 for TCM treatment.

On examination, she was found to be an old female with a fat physique, clear mind, dark tongue with whitish thick coating and wiry slippery pulse. The blood pressure was $22/12.5/kPa$,cholesterol 7.5mmol/L, triglyceride 2.4mmol/L, blood sugar 9.6mmol/L, the urine sugar $+++$ and the ketone in urine(-) . The electrocardiography revealed T:I. avl, V_{4-6} was lower and flat and ST segment shifted $0.5-1mm$ downwards. As a result, the diagnosis was made as diabetes complicated by hypertention and coronary heart diseases with angina pectoris. In the view of TCM, the disease was

162

caused by accumulation of phlegm-dampness in the interior which lead to failure of the clear to ascend and the turbid to descend. Because the coagulated blood obstructed the vessles, cardiac pain radiating to the back arised.

Therapeutic method: Dissolving phlegm and removing obstruction of the vessels, assisted by activating blood flow to relieve pain.

Prescription:

① Ban Xia(Rhizoma Pinelliae) 10g, Bai Zhu(Rhizoma Atractylodis Macrocephalae) 12g, Tian Ma(Rhizoma Gastridiae, to be decocted first) 15g, Fu Ling(Poria) 15g, Shi Chang Pu(Rhizoma Acori Graminei) 12g, Zhu Ru(Caulis Bambusae in Taeniam) 12g, Chen Pi (Pericarpium Citri Reticulatae) 9g, Dan Shen(Radix Salviae Miltiorrhizae) 30g, Chuan Xiong(Rhizoma Ligustici Chuanxiong) 12g, Gua Lou (Fructus Trichosanthis) 15g, Zhi Ke (Fructus Aurantii)9g and Gan Cao (Radix Glycyrrhizae) 6g, to be decocted in water for oral dose.

② Xiaoke Wan(Pills for Treating Diabetes), 10 pills each time, three times daily.

③ Xiaoke Ping(Tablets for Treating Diabetes), 8 tablets each time, three times daily.

After fiftcen doses continuous administration of the recipe, dizziness, headache and vertigo were alleviated, which indicated that Compound Hypotensor and Nitroglycerin could be stopped. Then more 40 doses of the above recipe with modifications in accordance with symptoms were administered which relieved markedly the symptoms. On reexaminations, the blood sugar was 5. 2mmol/L, the cholesterol 4. 9 mmol/L, the triglyceride 0. 8mmol/L, the urine glucose negative, and blood pressure 20/10 kPa. The ECG showed that S-T segment shifts downwards slightly. Then decoction of Chinese herbs was stopped but Xiaoke Wan (Pills for Treating Diabetes, which was to be taken 5 pills each time, twice daily, and Xiaoke Ping, to be taken 6 tablets each time, twice daily, were continued to fortify the therapeutic effects. He was also advised to do more exercise and control his diet well to prevent aggravation of the diabetes.

Case 3.

Liu was a 66 year-old male official clerk who was found to have diabetes three years ago. When he came to our hospital on March 5th, 1990, he complaint of oppressed feeling over the chest, shortness of breath, lassitude, dizziness, vertigo, frequent stabbling pain in the precardiac region which radiates to the left shoulder, induced by exertion and relieved by rest or taking Huo Xin Dan(Bolus for Promoting Flow of Blood in the Heart Vessel). But he had not obvious polyphagia, polydipsia, polyuria and emaciation.

On examination, he was found to be an old male with clear consciousness, lustreless face, red tongue with little coating, wiry and thready pulse; blood pressure was $20/14/kPa$, ECG showed that the V_{4-6} shifted downwards and the $T: V_{1-3}$ was conversed and V_{4-6} was in a lower and flat level. He had a blood sugar of 9. 8mmol/L, blood cholesterol of 7. 2mmol/L, and triglyceride of 1. 6 mmol/L. His urine glucose was $(++)$ and the ketone in urine was not found.

Diagnosis: diabetes complicated by hypertension and coronary heart disease in the view of Western medicine; deficiency of both qi and yin complicated by obstruction of the heart blood in the view of TCM.

Therapeutic method: Invigorating qi and nourishing yin, supported by promoting circulation of blood and removing blood stasis.

Prescription:

① Huang Qi (Radix Astragali seu Hedysari) 20g, Dang Shen (Radix Codonopsis Pilosulae) 15g, Mai Dong(Radix Ophiopogonis) 15g, Wu Wei Zi (Fructus Schisandrae) 9g, Dan Shen(Radix Salviae Miltiorrhizae) 30g, Ge Gen(Radix Puerariae) 15g, Chuan Xiong (Rhizoma Chuanxiong) 12g, Sha Shen (Radix Adenophorae Strictae) 15g, Yu Zhu (Rhizoma Polygonati Odorati), Yuan Hu (Rhizoma Corydalis) 9g, Hua Fen(Radix Trichosanthis) 30g, Zhi

164

Mu(Rhizoma Anemarrhenae), 12g, Gan Cao(Radix Glycyrrhizae) 6g, to be decocted in water for oral dose, one dose each day.

② Xiaoke Tablet, to be taken 8 tablets each time, three times daily.

③ Caculus Bolus for Lowering Blood Pressure, to be taken one bolus each time, three trimes daily.

During the administration of the above drugs, the Chinese formula had been modified in accordance with changes of the patient's symptoms, tongue and pulse. Reexamination performed after 30 doses had been administered indicated that all his symptoms had disappeared; the ECG showed no obvious pathologic change, the blood sugar was 5. 2mmol/L, the blood cholesterol was 5. 2mmol/L and the triglyceride was 1. 0mmol/L. No urine glucose was found. He was then instructed to do more exercise, control diet well and keep on taking Xiaoke Ping, 6 tablets each time and twice daily to fortify the therapeutic effects and prevent the blood glucose from rising again.

7. 3 Diabetic retinal lesion

In recent years, cases of diabetes died of ketoacidosis and infection have been reduced markedly as a result of the invention of insulin and the wide application of antibiotics. Consequently, complications of the cardiovascular system have become the main cause of death, which accounts for approximately 70-80% of it. With the increasing incidence of diabetes and the prolongation the patients' lives, various disorders of the small and large vessels secondary to diabetes are bringing about more danger to the patients. Of the disorders, diabetic retinal lesion has become one of the most common and severe disorder of the micrangium. It was reported that about 50% of the diabetes was complicated by retinal lesion, which would cause such severe consequence as blindness and serve as one of the four diseases(senile degeneration of retina, diabetic retinal lesion, glaucoma and senile cataract)responsible for blindness. The mechanism is still not clearly known. Most doctors believes that the pathologic changes of the optical fundus may be related to the microangipathic lesion complicated with formation of microthrombus in the retinal microcirculation, the hypercoagulation, hyperviscosity and hyperaccumulation of the blood in diabetic patients. Abnormality of the vascular wall and that of the blood interfere with each other, forming a vicious circle in which they act as both the cause and result and finally result in the retinal lesion. As the mechanism is not clear enough, there is still no special therapy for the disease implemented in Western medicine.

According to TCM, the retinal lesion secondary to diabetes is ascribed to yin deficiency and dryness-heat, the basic pathogenesis of diabetes, and the subsequent failure of qi to be carried and the injury of vital qi by the dry-heat, which exist a long time and cause the combination of yin deficiency, dry-heat and qi deficiency. As a result, flow of blood in the optical vessels is impeded or the blood in the vessels is extravasated, leading to stagnation of blood in the optical fundus. Therefore, blood stasis or extravasation after rupture of the vessles are the main pathogenesis of the diabetic retinal lesion. If no timely treatment is given, the bleeding may occur repeatedly and produce macula, which is the main cause of blindness. The key to the treatment, therefore, lies in controlling the further development of the disease and preventing the occurrence of blindness. TCM treatment is usually performed on the basis of the disease identification and syndrome identification by dividing the disease in several types. By now, there have been a lot of reports on cases treated with TCM, the results have showed that TCM treatment could control the further development of the disease but could not cure it. For this reason, therapeutic methods should be formulated based on the different pathologic changes of the optical fundus detected through modern equipment and the various manifestations of diabetes in the course of treatment. The types and treatments are as follows:

7. 3. 1 Type of yin deficiency and dryness-heat

Main manifestations: Polydipsia, polyorexia, blurred vision, reddened tongue with yellow and dry coating, thready rapid or full rapid pulse which is forceless on heavy pressure.

Therapeutic method: Clearing away heat, moistening dryness and nourishing yin to improve eyesight.

Prescription: Huang Lian (Rhizoma Coptidis) 10g, Shi Gao (Gypsum Fibrosum) 30g, Hua Fen (Radix Trichosanthis) 30g, Mai Dong (Radix Ophiopogonis) 12g, Nu Zhen Zi (Fructus Ligustici Lucidi) 12g, Sheng Di (Radix Rehmanniae) 15g, Xuan Shen (Radix Scrophulariae) 15g, Gu Jing Cao (Flos Eriocauli) 15g, to be decocted in water for oral use.

7. 3. 2 Type of deficiency of both the liver-yin and the kidney-yin

Main manifestations: Polydipsia, soreness and weakness of the loins and knees, feverish sensation over the palms, soles and chest, frequent and profuse urine, dizziness, blurred vision, reddened tongue with little coating, and thready rapid pulse.

Therapeutic method: Clearing away heat from the liver to improve the eyesight, nourishing both the liver and the kidney.

Prescription: Gou Qi (Fructus Lycii) 12g, Shan Yu Rou (Fructus Cornu) 12g, Ju Hua (Flos Chrysanthemi) 10g, Mu Dan Pi (Cortex Moutan Radicis) 10g, Sheng Di (Radix Rehmanniae) 15g, Shan Yao (Rhizoma Dioscoreae) 15g, Ze Xie (Rhizoma ALismatis) 15g, Fu Ling (Poria), Gu Jing Cao (Flos Eriocauli) 15g, Cao Jue Ming (Semen Cassiae) 30g, to be decocted in water for oral dose.

7. 3. 3 Type of deficiency of both the lung-yin and the kidney-yin

Main manifestations: Dry mouth and throat, severe thirst, frequent urination, lassitude, blurred vision, red tongue with litte fluid, thready and rapid pulse.

Therapeutic method: Clearing away heat, moistening the lung, nourishing the kidney and improving eyesight.

Prescription: Tian Dong (Radix Asparagi) 12g, Mai Dong (Radix Ophiopogonis) 12g, Zhi Mu (Rhizoma Anemarrhenae) 12g, Sheng

Di (Radix Rehmanniae) 12g, Xuan Shen (Radix Scrophulariae) 12g, Shi Hu(Herba Dendrobii) 12g, Sha Shen (Radix Adenophorae Strictae) 15g, Ge Gen(Radix Puerariae) 15g, Huang Qi (Radix Astragali seu Hedysari) 30g, Hua Fen (Radix Trichosanthis) 30g, Huang Lian(Rhizoma Coptidis) 10g, to be decocted in water for oral use.

7. 3. 4 Deficiency of both the kidney-yin and the kidney-yang

Main manifestations: Frequent urination, aversion to cold and cold limbs, impotence in male, soreness and weakness of the loins and knees, blurred vision, or even blindness, pale tongue with whitish coating, and deep thready and forceless pulse.

Therapeutic method: Nourishing the kidney and warming up yang.

Prescription: Fu Zi(Radix Aconiti) 6g, Rou Gui(Cortex Cinnamomi) 6g, Sheng Di(Radix Rehmanniae) 15g, Shan Yao(Rhizoma Dioscoreae) 15g, Shan Yu Rou (Fructus Corni) 15g, Ze Xie(Rhizoma Alismatis) 15g, Fu Ling(Poria) 15g, Dan Pi(Cortex Moutan Radicis) 9g, Huang Qi(Radix Astragali seu Hedysari) 30g, Dang Shen(Radix Codonopsis Pilosula) 15g, Gou Qi Zi(Fructus Lycii) 15g, Ju Hua(Flos Achrysanthemi) 9g, to be decocted in water for oral use.

Modifications in accordance with the symptoms:

① In the case of bleeding from the optical fundus at the early stage, the therapeutic method is to cool blood to stop bleeding, supplement qi and nourish yin. The drugs selected to be added to the recipe are: Sheng Di (Radix Rehmanniae), Dan Pi (Cortex Moutan Radicis), Xian He Cao(Herba Agrimoniae), Bai Mao Gen(Rhizoma Imperatae), Da Ji (Herba seu Radix Cirsii Faponici), Xiao Ji(Herba Cephalanoploris), Nu Zhen Zi (Fructus Ligustri Lucidi), Han Lian Cao(Herba Ecliptae), San Qi Fen(Powder of Radix Notoginseng), etc.

② In the case of prolonged accumulation of the extravasated

168

blood, the treatment should be supported by promoting circulation of blood and removing blood stasis. To the recipe, the following drugs can be added deliberately: Dan Shen (Radix Salviae Miltiorrhizae), Chi Shao (Radix Paeoniae Rubra), Hong Hua (Flos Carthami), Ze Lan (Herba Lycopi), Yu Jin (Radix Curcumae), Tu Si Zi (Semen Cuscutae), Han Lian Cao (Herba Ecliptae), Hua Lei Shi (Ophicalcitum), Pu Huang (Pollen Typhae), etc.

The bleeding may occur repeatedly because of the impairment of the vessels, so administration of blood flow-promoting and blood stasis-removing drugs alone must be with great care. In most cases, drugs arresting bleeding by removing blood stasis should be adopted in combination under strict observation to avoid any unexpected crisis.

③ At the restoration stage, the extravasated blood is mostly absorbed or becomes ecchymosis or small nodules. Therefore, the treatment should be aimed at invigorating qi, promoting flow of blood, softening hardness and dissipiting masses. Drugs to be adopted are: Huang Qin (Radix Scutellariae) 30g, Cang Zhu (Rhizoma Atractylodis) 30g, Shan Yao (Rhizoma Dioscoreae) 15g, Xuan Shen (Radix Scrophulariae) 15g, Tu Si Zi (Semen Cuscutae) 15g, Nu Zhen Zi (Fructus Ligustri Lucidi), Hong Hua (Flos Carthami) 15g, Bei Mu (Bulbus Fritillariae Thunbergii) 12g, Chuan Xiong (Rhizoma Ligustici Chuanxiong) 12g, Mu Li (Concha Ostreae) 30g, Hai Ge Fen (Geckonaidiae) 30g, to be decocted in water for oral dose.

For cases with well-controlled blood sugar and urine glucose and mild manifestations, only one formula with modifications can be applied. Ingredients of the formula are: Huang Qi (Radix Astragali seu Hedysari), Shan Yao (Rhizoma Dioscoreae), Cang Zhu (Rhizoma Atractylodis), Sheng Di (Radix Rehmanniae), Shi Hu (Herba Dendrobii), Gou Qi Zi (Fructus Lycii), Ge Gen (Radix Puerariae), Dan Shen (Radix Salviae Miltiorrhizae), Tu Si Zi (Semen Cuscutae), Chuan Xiong (Rhizoma Ligusttici Chuanxiong), Gu Jing Cao (Flos Eriocauli), Cao Jue Ming (Semen Cassiae), Ju Hua (Flos Achrysanthemi), Bei Mu(Bulbus Fritillariae), Kun Bu(Thallus Laminariae seu Ekloniae), Xian He Cao(Herba Agrimoniae). This formula aims at benefiting qi, nourishing yin, removing blood stasis and dissolving masses to improve eyesight.

7. 3. 5 Case Study

Zhu was a 50 -year old female who had been ill with diabetes for 8 years and had progressive blurred vision for 3 yeras. Before her visit, she had been taking oral glybenzcyclamide(three tablets daily) and controlling her diet,so her blood sugar had been kept within 11. $2-16.5$ mmol/L,the urine glucose $++-+$,and her urine ketone had been (−). On her visit, she had polydipsia, polyphagia, frequent and profuse urine, dizziness, vertigo, blurred vision, dry stool, red tongue with little coating and thready rapid pulse. In the past several days, the blurred vision was gradually aggravated. Ophthalmic examination revealed that $^{1.0}_{1.0}$ her external eyes were normal, but the cortical opacity and heterogeneity of the anterior and posterior capsules of the bilateral lens were found. Fundus of the both eyes showed normal optic disc, scattered blood spot, extensive exudate and botuliform venous engorgement on the retina. So she was diagnosed as having diabetic retinal lesion of simple type III on both eyes, complicated by cataract. Then she was prescribed:

① Qiju Dihuang Wan(Rehammania Root Decoction with Wolfberry Fruit and Chrysanthemum Flower)with modification, ingredients of which were:

Gou Qi Zi(Fructus Lycii) 12g, Ju Hua(Flos Chrysanthemi) 9g, Sheng Di (Radix Rehmanniae) 15g, Mu Dan Pi(Cortex Moutan Radicis) 9g, Shan Yu Rou (Fructus Corni) 12g, Shan Yao(Rhizoma Dioscoreae) 15g, Ze Xie(Rhizoma Alismatis) 15g, Xuan Shen (Radix Scrophulariae) 12g, Bai Mao Gen (Rhizoma Imperatae) 30g, Han Lian Cao(Herba Ecliptae) 30g, Cang Zhu(Rhizoma Atractylodis) 20g, Gu Jing Cao(Flos Eriocali), and Jing Jie Tan(Spica Schizonepetae, calcinated), to be decocted in water for oral administration, one dose daily.

② Diamicron, to be taken 80 mg each time, three times daily.

Half a mouth later, the patient came for consultation again and complaint of an alleviation of the diabetic symptoms with reduced amount of urine and clearer vision than before. Blood glucose was 11. 2mmol/L and the urine glucose was(＋＋). Optical examination showed $\frac{4.3}{5.2}$, but the condition of the bilateral cystalline lens remained the same as before, the fresh bleeding from the retina was fundamentally stopped and the exudate was reduced. Then with 12g of Nu Zhen Zi(Fructus Ligustri Lucudi) added, the previous formula was prescribed again for further continuous use. The formula was administered with modification for 4 months, then she underwent a reexamination, which showed that the blood glucose reduced to 8. 4 mmol/L and the urine glucose, (＋). Optical examination was $\frac{4.5}{5.3}$, no fresh bleeding was found and part of the remote extravasated blood had been absorbed and the exudate had become remote. Diabetic retinal lesion is indeed a severe complication which often develops further to cause blindness if no active treatment is given. Therefore, it is imperative to diagnose and treat the disease earlier so as to lower the blindness rate. To reduce blood sugar vigorously and prevent its fluctuation with both Western and Chinese herbal medicine can improve evidently the therapeutic effect and control the development of the disease, thus the patients' emotion can be relaxed and their suffering alleviated.

7. 4 Diabetes complicated with ketosis

When the administration of insulin is stopped or the dose is not adequate in the treatment of insulin-dependent diabetes, or various stresses happen to those with non-insulin-dependent diabetes, the disturbance of metabolism will be aggravated, the fat decompose more rapidly, and the ketone accumulate and the blood ketone may be so high as to be 2mmol/L more than the normal value as a result of its

171

increased production. This condition is called ketonemia, or diabetic ketonemia clinically. When metabolic acidosis occurs as a result of the accumulation of ketone, it is named diabetic ketoacidosis. And if the ketoacidosis develops coma, it is termed diabetic ketoacidosis coma. Diabetes complicated with ketosis is a severe and emergent condition, to which early prevention and treatment must be given.

There are few reports on the TCM treatment of diabetic ketosis on the textbooks and other literatures. However, TCM treatment is often applied clinically and can bring about rather satisfactory effects. According to the results of laboratory tests and the patients' clinical manifestations, proper measures can be taken by combining the Western diagnosis and the syndrome identification of TCM based on the fundamental principles for diagnosis and treatment of TCM. For diabetes complicated by ketosis, TCM treatment can be applied to the following three conditions.

7. 4. 1 Early stage of diabetic ketosis

When the urine ketone is kept positive or becomes positive suddenly without the manifestations of ketoacidosis such as coma or shock, adjustment of the dose of the oral antihypoglycemic agents and the application of the decoction of Chinese herbs can be effective. Insulin therapy is not necessary. In most cases, the ketone in the urine will become negative after 6-10 doses of Chinese herbs are administered and further application of the decoction can fortify the therapeutic effect, preventing the reccurrence of the urine ketone. The main ingredients of the formula to be selected are:

Hua Fen(Radix Trichosanthis) 30g, Sheng Shi Gao(Gypsum Fibrosum) 30g, Jin Yin Hua(Fios Lonicrae) 30g, Pu Gong Ying(Herba Taraxaci) 30g, Long Gu (Os Draconis) 30g, Mu Li(Concha Ostreae) 30g, Huang Lian(Rhizoma Coptidis) 15g, Zhi Mu(Rhizoma Anemarrhenae) 15g, Huang Qin(Radix Scutellariae) 10g, Mu Dan Pu (Cortex Moutan Radicis) 20g, Sheng Di (Radix Rehmanniae) 20g, Xuan Shen(Radix Scrophulariae) 20g, Cang Zhu(Rhizoma A-

172

tractylodis) 20g, Rou Gui(Cortex Cinnamomi) 3g, to be decocted in water for oral dose.

In this formula, Hua Fen, Zhi Mu, Sheng Di and Dan Pi are used to nourish yin, clear away heat and promote the production of the body fluid. As the assistant drugs, Sheng Shi Gao, Huang Qin and Huang Lian are used to clear away heat and purge fire, Long Gu and Mu Li to suppress yang and nourish yin, Cang Zhu and Xuan Shen to strengthen the spleen and nourish the kidney and lower the blood sugar. As the guiding drug, Rou Gui functions to induce the fire to flow downward to the kidney. Jin Yin Hua and Pu Gong Ying are used here to clear away heat and remove toxic materials to prevent infection and treat the induction pathologic changes.

Modifications in accordance with symptoms:

① For cases with obvious infection, the formula should be modified in accordance with different causes and different affected parts. For the cases due to sores, add Di Ding(Herba Corydalis Bungenae), Ye Ju Hua(Flos Chrysanthemi), Chi Shao(Radix Poaeniae Rubra), etc.; for the cases caused by toothache or periodonitis, add Huai Niu Xi (Radix Achyranthis Bidentatae), Bai Zhi (Radix Angelicae Dahuricae), Xi Xin(Herba Asari); for the cases due to affection of exogenous wind-cold, add Qiang Huo (Rhizoma seu Radix Notopetrygii), Su Ye (Folium Perillae) and Fang Feng (Radix Ledebouriellae); for cases due to affection of exogenous wind-heat, add Chai Hu(Radix Bupleuri), Ge Gen(Radix Puerariae), Da Qing Ye (Folium Isatidis), Ban Lan Gen(Radix Isatidis), etc.

② In the case of proteinuria, add Chuan Duan(Radix Dipsari), Bai Hua She She Cao (Herba Hedyotis Diffusae), Chan Tui (Periostracum Cicadae), and Yi Mu Cao(Herba Leonuri).

③ For the cases complicated with urinary infection, add deliberately Di Ding(Herba Corydalis Bungenae), Di Fu Zi(Fructus Kochia), Huang Bai (Cortex Phellodendri), Bai Mao Gen (Rhizoma Imperatae), etc.

④ For cases with persistent high ketone, add Ban Lan Gen(Radix Isatidis), Da Qing Ye(Folium Isatidis),Zi Cao(Radix Arnebiae)and Rou Gui(Cortex Cinnamomi).

⑤ For cases with pulmonary tuberculosis, add Huang Jing(Rhizoma Polygonati), Bai Bu(Radix Stemonae), Jiang Can(Bombyx Batriticatus), Bai Ji(Rhizoma Bletillae), etc.

⑥ For cases with evident blood stasis, add Dan Shen(Radix Salviae Miltiorrhizae), Chi Shao(Radix Paeoniae Rubra), Tao Ren(Semen Persicae), Hong Hua(Flos Carthami), Yi Mu Cao(Herba Leonuri), Di Long(Lumbricus), etc. If the cases are originally complicated by coronary heart disease marked by obstruction of the heart vessel or by hemiplegia, more drugs for activating blood flow and removing blood stasis should be added.

⑦ For cases with hyperthyroidism and thyroid enlargement, drugs dissipating masses and relieving the thyroid enlargement should be added apart from those replenishing qi, nourishing yin and calming the mind. The added drugs are: Wa Leng Zi(Concha Arcae), Mu Li (Concha Ostreae), Ji Nei Jin(Endothelium Corneum Gigeriae), San Leng(Rhizoma Sparganii), E Zhu (Rhizoma Zedoariae), Xia Ku Cao(Spica Prunellae), Hai Zao(Sargassum), Kun Bu(Thallus Eckloniae), etc.

⑧ For cases with heat transformed from accumulated turbid-dampness in the interior, marked by red togue with yellow and greasy coating, soft and rapid pulse, the treatment should be assisted by clearing away heat, inducing diuresis to remove turbid-dampness. So, add Huo Xiang(Herba Agastachis), Pei Lan(Herba Eupatorii), Sha Ren (Fructus Amomi), Bai Kou Ren(Semen Amomi Cardamomi)and Cao Dou Kou(Semen Alpiniae Katsumadai) to the formula to eliminate ketone by removing stagnated qi and dissolving the turbid-yin.

7. 4. 2 Stage of diabetic ketoacidosis

First aid must be given to those with diabetic ketoacidosis marked by shock and coma. Chinese drugs such as Zixue Dan (a Chinese

174

patent drug from *Presciptions of Peaceful Benevolent Dispensary*) may be chosen to clear away heat, detoxicate, relieve convulsion and induce resuscitation by filling and nasal feeding. Zhi Bao Dan(also from the *Prescriptions of Peaceful Benevolent Dispensary*) can also be adopted by taking 3—5 boluses with decoction of Ren Shen(Radix Ginseng) to dissolve the turbid substances, restore consciousness and induce resuscitation. The above drugs are indicative for coma and delirium caused by inward attack of pathogens on the pericardium or by obstruction of the accumulated heat in the interior. As the pathogenesis of the diabetic ketoacidosis lies in stagnation of dry-heat and toxic materials in the blood, the ensuing impairment of yin and the exhaustion of both yin and yang, and the failure of the lucid yang to ascend due to accumulation of toxic heat and turbid substances, coma and delirium occur as a result. For such cases, the three precious drugs, namely, Zi Xue Dan, Zhi Bao Dan and Su He Xiang Wan, should be given as first aid.

7. 4. 3 Stage of ketoacidosis without coma or the ketoacidosis after emergent treatment

Positive treatment should be continued to prevent the occurrence of coma due to ketoacidosis or recurrence of the ketoacidosis after emergent treatment. At this stage, the unexhausted dry-heat and the stagnated turbid-qi impair both qi and yin, leading to coexistence of both yin deficiency and dry-heat. Therefore, this stage is usually identified as a syndrome deficiency in origin and excess in superfiality, or that of deficiency complicated with excess, with stagnation of the turbid-qi as the secondary condition and impairment of both qi and yin as the fundamental. The treatment should be aimed at clearing away heat, removing toxic materials and lowering down the turbid to eliminate dryness-heat and dissolve turbid yin substances, assisted by supplementing qi, nourishing yin, and harmonizing blood, to strengthen the vital qi and the consolidate the constitution. By means of treating both the origin and the superfiality, the dry-heat can be eliminated,

175

the blood flow and the distribution of the body fluid restored to normal and the stagnated turbid-qi dissolved. As a result, qi and yin can be supplemented.

Continuous use of Chinese herbs can promote the earlier restoration of the strength and prevent the ketone in the urine from occurring again, which can help stablize the disease and regulate the dosage of the Western drugs as well as insulin.

Ingredients of the commonly used formula are: Huang Lian (Rhizoma Coptidis) 15g, Huang Qin (Radix Scutellariae) 15g, Zhi Zi (Fructus Gardeniae) 10g, Sheng Di (Radix Rehmanniae) 20g, Xuan Shen (Radix Scrophulariae) 20g, Shan Yao (Rhizoma Dioscoreae) 20g, Cang Zhu (Rhizoma Atractylodis) 24g, Huang Qi (Radix Astragali seu Hedysari) 30g, Hua Fen (Radix Trichosanthis) 30g, Chi Shao (Radix Paeoniae Rubra) 15g, Pei Lan (Herba Eupatorii) 12g, and Da Huang (Radix et Rhizoma Rhei, to be added to the decoction later) 10g, to be decocted in water for oral use.

This formula functions to supplement qi and nourish yin, clear away heat, harmonize blood, strengthen the spleen and dissolve the turbid. Clinically, stresses may be placed on some of these functions, depending on severity of the illness and relation between the excess and deficiency and that between the fundamentals and superficials. For cases with excessive pathogenic factors, the treatment should be directed at treating the superficials first by clearing away heat, harmonizing blood, lowering down the turbid to treat ketoacidosis. When the pathogens are expelled, the treatment should be aimed at strenthening the vital qi and consolidating the constitution by tonifying both the spleen and the kidney or by tonifying qi and nourishing yin, so that both the fundamentals and the superficials are treated.

Modifications in accordance with symptoms and signs:

① For cases with severe polydipsia, add Sheng Shi Gao (Gypsum Fibrosum), Zhi Mu (Rhizoma Anemarrhenae) and Hai Ge Fen (Geckonidae).

② For cases with nausea and vomiting, add Chen Pi(Pericarpium Citri Reticulatae), Ban Xia(Rhizoma Pinelliae), and Zhu Ru(Caulis Bombusae in Taeniam), or replace the original formula with Huanglian Wendan Tang (Coptis Decoction for Clearing Away Heat from the Gallbladder).

③For cases with blurred vision, add Gou Qi Zi(Fructus Lycii), Ju Hua (Flos Chrysanthemi), Cao Jue Ming(Semen Cassiae), Chong Wei Zi(Fructus Leonuri) and Shi Hu(Herba Dendrobii).

④ For cases with frequent urination with profuse urine at night, add Fu Pen Zi(Fructus Rubi), Tu Si Zi(Semen Cuscutae), Wu Bei Zi(Galla Chinensis), Jin Ying Zi(Fructus Rosae Laevigatae), etc.

⑤ For cases with proteinuria, add Chuan Duan(Radix Dipsaci), Bai Hua She She Cao(Herba Hedyotis Diffusae) and increase the dosage of Huang Qi (Radix Astragali seu Hedysari)and Shan Yao (Rhizoma Dioscoreae).

⑥ For cases with sleepiness, add Shi Chang Pu(Rhizoma Acori Graminei), Yuan Zhi(Radix Polygalae) and Yu Jin(Radix Curcumae) to restore resuscitation.

⑦ For cases with hypertension, marked by headache and dizziness, add Tian Ma(Rhizoma Gastrodiae), Gou Teng(Ramulus Uncariae cum Uncis) and Long Chi(Dens Draconis).

⑧ For cases marked by yin deficiency, add Shi Hu(Herba Dendrobii), Yu Zhu (Rhizoma Polygonati Odorati), Mai Dong (Radix Ophiopogonis), Wu Wei Zi (Fructus Schisandrae), Tai Zi Shen (Radix Pseudostellariae), etc. , to supplement and nourish yin.

This formula is mainly composed of bitter and cold drugs. So, if ketone in the urine is removed and patient's contion is stable, the drugs bitter in taste and cold in nature should be reduced from the formula lest they impair the stomach. At this time, drugs and formula can be applied according to the common rule of administration of drugs for diabetes. The patient should be advised to receive treatment

177

positively, continue medication and the insulin treatment, in order to avoid recurrence of ketosis and aggravation of the disease. Critical patients should be hospitalized and the induction factor must be removed so that they can recovery from their disease earlier.

7. 4. 4 Case Study

Li was a 35-year old male who had been ill with diabetes for 3 years. He had been treated with oral glybenzcyclamide by taking 6 tablets each time. When he came for medical care, he had polydipsia, polyuria, emaciation, lassitude, sleepiness, listlessness, disinclination to talk, numbness of the limbs, nausea, poor appetite,dry stool, dark tongue with little fluid, yellow coating and wiry slippery pulse. The laboratory tests showed that the fasting blood sugar was 20. 3 mmol/L, the urine glucose (+ + + +), and the ketone in urine (+ +). Then the diagnosis was made as diabetic ketosis in the view of Western medicine and yin deficiency and dryness-heat complicated by exuberance of toxic heat in the interior and impairment of both qi and yin in the view of TCM.

Therapeutic method: Clearing away heat, removing toxic materials, tonifying qi and nourishing yin.

Prescription: Xiao Tong Tang(Decoction for Eliminating Ketone) with modification,ingredients of which are:

Huang Lian (Rhizoma Coptidis) 9g, Zhi Zi (Fructus Gardeniae) 10g, Xuan Shen(Radix Scrophulariae) 30g, Sheng Di Huang(Radix Rehmanniae) 15g, Tian Hua Fen (Radix Trichosanthis) 30g, Shan Yao(Rhizoma Dioscoreae) 15g, Cang Zhu (Rhizoma Atractylodis) 12g, Fu Ling(Poria) 15g, Pei Lan(Herba Eupatorii) 12g, Zhu Ru (Caulis Bombusae in Taeniam) 10g, Huang Qi(Radix Astragali seu Hedysari) 30g, Da Huang(Radix et Rhizoma Rhei, to be added to the decoction later) 6g, and Gan Cao(Radix Glycyrrhizae) 6g, to be decocted in water for oral use,one dose daily.

The patient was also instructed to take glybencyclimide, 2. 5 mg each time, three times daily.

After three doses of the formula were administered, the patient complaint of alleviation of thirst, increase of the strength of the lower limbs, better spirit, and one bowel movement with soft stool daily. His tongue and pulse were the same as before, and the urine glucose was found to be $+++$ and the ketone in the urine $+$. Then the original formula was continued until his symptoms were greatly alleviated after more 12 doses were administered. His nausea and vomiting disappeared and he had a normal diet with 250g of stable food (flour) daily. Laboratory test revealed that the blood sugar at an empty stomach was 15.7 mmol/L, liver function was normal, the glucose in the urine was $++$, and the ketone in the urine became negative. As a result, formula with the function of nourishing the kidney, strengthening the spleen, nourishing blood and activating the blood flow was prescribed to fortify the therapeutic effects and treat diabetes continuously. Ketone in the urine was not found in a half-a-year follow-up.

7.5 Diabetes complicated by acromelic necrosis (diabetic foot)

Patients with diabetes often present various kinds of skin lesions, of which the most commonly encountered are such acute infections as boils, intumescence and carbuncles. At the later stage, necrosis of the endings of the extremities, marked by infection and necrosis of the fingers, toes or the whole foot, often occurs as a result of malnutrition of the peripheral nerves and the disorders of the microcirculation.

Diabetic foot is a morbid state marked by loss of sense due to nervous disorders and infection secondary to ischemia, which may be induced by improper changes of cold and heat, infection after traumatic injury, impeded flow of blood resulting in obstruction of the local vessels and the ensuing ischemia and necrosis, local compressing resulting in small wound, and improper management of the corn leading to impairment of the skin. If sensory decline or disappearance occurs simultaneously and is not noticed promptly, the wound may become larger and cause necrosis. When severe infection or necrosis presents, the treatment will become very difficult and debility or even death may ensue.

Acromelic necrosis in diabetes is named Tuo Ju in TCM. It is mostly caused by the stagnation of fire in the zang-fu organs resulting from deficient yin faling to control the fire, or by affection of exogenous toxic cold and dampness which leads to disharmony between the nutritive qi and the defensive qi and the subsequent stagnation of both qi and blood. The treatment should be aimed at removing toxic materials to relieve pain, promoting blood circulation and removing blood stasis. For cases with more dampness-cold, drugs warming channels and expelling cold should be added; and for cases with deficiency of both qi and blood, drugs supplementing qi and tonifying blood should be used in combination. The commonly used formulas in the clinic are: Jiedu Jisheng Tang (Decoction for Detoxicating and Benefiting Patients, from *Orthodox Manual of Surgery*), which consists of Chuan Xiong (Rhizoma Ligustici Chuanxiong), Dang Gui (Radix Angelicae Sinensis), Huang Bai (Cortex Phellodendrii), Zhi Mu (Rhizoma Anemarrhenae), Tian Hua Fen (Radix Trichosanthis), Jin Yin Hua (Flos Lonicerae), Mai Dong (Radix Ophiopogonis), Yuan Zhi (Radix Polygalae), Chai Hu (Radix Bupleuri), Huang Qin (Radix Scutellariae), Hong Hua (Flos Carthami), Sheng Ma (Rhizoma Cimicifugae), Niu Xi (Radix Achyranthis Bidentatae), and Gan Cao (Radix Glycyrrhizae); Simiao Yongan Tang (Decoction of Four Wonderful Drugs for Detoxicating and Removing Blood Stasis, from *New Compilation of Proved Formulas*) which is composed of: Jin Yin Hua (Flos Lonicerae), Xuan Shen (Radix Scrophulariae), Dang Gui (Radix Angelicae Sinensis) and Gan Cao (Radix Glycyrrhizae) ; Yanghe Tang (Decoction for Warming Yang, from *Complete Works of Diagnosis and Treatment for Surgical Diseases*) which contains: Shu Di (Radix Rehmanniae Praeparata), Bai Jie Zi (Semen Sinapis Alba), Lu Jiao Jiao (Colla Cornus Cervi), Rou Gui (Cortex Cinnamomi),

180

Ma Huang (Herba Ephedrae), Pao Jiang (Rhizoma Zingiberis Praeparata), and Gan Cao(Radix Glycyrrhizae), etc. More satisfactory effects can be obtained if external application is adopted in combination to control the blood sugar and infection positively on the basis of the diagnosis of disease according to Western medicine and the diagnosis of syndrome according to TCM.

7. 5. 1 Type of yin deficiency and heat exuberance complicated by blood stasis

Main manifestations: Pain of bilateral or unilateral leg with a dark purple color, black toes or small erosions, absence of obvious polydipsia, polyphagia and polyuria, elevation of blood sugar and urine glucose, accompanied with blurred vision, red tongue with little coating or dotted with ecchymosis or petechia, thready and hesitant pulse.

Therapeutic method: Nourishing yin to clear away heat, supplementing qi and removing blood stasis.

Prescription: Zhi Mu (Rhizoma Anemarrhenae) 12g, Sheng Di (Radix Rehmanniae) 12g, Huang Bai (Cortex Phellodendri) 10g, Shan Yao(Rhizoma Dioscoreae) 15g, Fu Ling(Poria) 15g, Ze Xie (Rhizoma Alismatis) 15g, Mu Dan Pi(Cortex Moutan Radicis) 15g, Xuan Shen(Radix Scrophulariae) 15g, Cang Zhu(Rhizoma Atractylodis) 20g, Dang Gui(Radix Angelicae Sinensis) 20g, Jin Yin Hua (Flos Lonicerae) 30g, Dan Shen(Radix Salviae Miltiorrhizae) 30g, Huang Qi (Radix Astragali seu Hedysari) 30g, to be decocted in water for oral use.

Modifications in accordance with symptoms:

① For cases with damp gangrene, add Pu Gong Ying (Herba Taraxaci) 30g, Lian Qiao(Fructus Forsythiae)15g and increase the dosage of Jin Yin Hua(Flos Lonicerae)to 60g.

② For cases with dry gangrene, add Shui Zhi(Hirudo) 10g, Tao Ren (Semen Persicae) 10g and Hong Hua(Flos Carthami) 10g.

③ For cases with cold ending of extremeties with aversion to cold, add Gui Zhi(Ramulus Cinnamomi) 10g.

181

7. 5. 2 Type of blood stasis in the interior and obstruction of vessels

Main manifestations: Numbness of limbs, dark purple colour of the gangrene region which becomes pale when lying flat and even darker with plaque when drooping the leg, unbearable and fixed pain of the affected leg, dark purple tongue, and thready and hesitant pulse.

Therapeutic method: Promoting the blood flow and removing blood stasis, removing obstruction of the vessels and harmonizing blood.

Prescription: Dang Gui(Radix Angelicae Sinensis) 15g, Chi Shao (Radix Paeoniae Rubra) 15g, Chuan Xiong (Rhizoma Ligustici Chuanxiong) 20g, Dan Shen(Radix Salviae Miltiorrhizae) 30g, Ren Dong Teng(Caulis Lonicerae) 30g, Chuan Niu Xi(Radix Cyathulae) 30g, Hong Hua(Flos Carthami) 12g, Zhi Ru Xiang(Resina Olibani) 10g, Zhi Mo Yao(Myrrhae) 10g, Gan Cao(Radix Glycyrrhizae) 6g, to be decocted in water for oral dose.

Modification in accordance with symptoms:

① For cases with more dampness-heat, marked by thirst but with no desire for drinks, dark tongue with thick and greasy coating, add Cang Zhu (Rhizoma Atractylodis) 24g and Huang Bai(Cortex Phellondendri) 12g.

② For cases with obvious deficiency of qi, add Huang Qi(Radix Astragali seu Hedysari) 30—60g, Dang Shen(Radix Codonopsis Pilosula) 20—30g, and Bai Zhu(Rhizoma Atractylodis Macrocephalae) 15g.

③ For cases with severe yin deficiency, marked by dry mouth, thirst with desire for drinks, red tongue with little coating, add Sheng Di (Radix Rehmanniae) 15g, Mai Dong (Radix Ophiopogonis) 15g, Xuan Shen (Radix Scrophulariae) 15g, Sha Shen(Radix Adenophorae Strictae) 15g, and Hua Fen (Radix Trichosanthis) 30g.

④ For cases with severe pain, add Wu Gong (Scolopendra) 2 pieces, Jiang Can (Bambyx Batryticatus) 10g, Yuan Hu (Rhizoma Corydalis) 10g, Di Long (Lumbricus, stir-fried) 12g, to remove obstruction in the vessels, expel wind and alleviate pain.

⑤ For cases with ulceration, apply Leech Tincture to the affected part. For cases with unruptured wound, soak and wash the affected part with the decoction of Huoxue Zhitong San (Powder for Promoting Blood Flow and Relieving Pain, a formula developed in our hospital) to improve the therapeutic effects.

This formula contains blood flow-promoting and blood stasis-removing drugs such as Dang Gui (Radix Angelicae Sinensis), etc., which have the effects of improving the blood flow to the cardiac vessels, dilating the peripheral vessels and improving the peripheral circulation, thus it has the function of relieving vascular convulsion, accelerating the construction of the collateral circulation, subduing swelling and treating inflammation.

7. 5. 3 Type of deficiency of vital qi, blood stasis and accumulation of toxic heat in the interior

Main manifestations: Long duration of diabetes, aggravation of the gangrene, emaciation, lassitude, or even persistent high fever due to invasion of toxic heat into blood, or impairment of both qi and yin due to the accumulated toxic heat developing pus, red tongue with little coating, and thready rapid pulse.

Therapeutic method: Supporting the vital qi, removing blood stasis, promoting healing of wound and the regeneration of tissues, clearing away heat and removing toxic materials.

Prescription: Huang Qi (Radix Astragali seu Hedysari) 30g, Shan Yao (Rhizoma Dioscoreae) 30g, Xuan Shen (Radix Scophulariae) 30g, Hua Fen (Radix Trichosanthis) 30g, Hang Shao (Chinese Herbaceous Peony) 30g, Dan Shen (Radix Salviae Miltiorrhizae) 30g, Shan Yu Rou (Fructus Cornu) 20g, Chi Shao (Radix Poaeniae Rubra) 20g, Jin Yin Hua (Flos Lonicerae) 60g, Pu Gong Ying (Herba Taraxaci) 60g, Dan Pi(Cortex Moutan Radicis) 10g, Ye Ju Hua (Flos Chrysanthemi Indici) 15g, and Chan Yi (Periostracum Cicadae) 10g, to be decocted in water for oral use.

Combined therapies of both Western and Chinese medicine are required in the treatment of the disease at this stage, for the symptoms are usually more severe. On the one hand, the blood sugar must be well controlled, on the other hand, the infection must be treated positively with broad-spectrum antibiotics so that the patients' condition can be improved.

To sum up, for diabetes complicated with severe skin infection and diabetic gangrene of the extremities, TCM treatment should be performed based on that for Xiaoke syndrome and Tuo Ju with supporting the vital qi, removing blood stasis, clearing away heat and removing toxic materials as the basic principle. The drugs to be selected include:Huang Qi(Radix Astragali seu Hedysari), Dang Shen(Radix Codonopsis Pilosulae), Bai Zhu(Rhizoma Atractylodis Macrocephalae), Cang Zhu(Rhizoma Atractylodis), Xuan Shen(Radix Scrophulariae), Ze Xie(Rhizoma Alismatis), Ze Lan(Herba Lycopi),Huang Bai (Cortex Phellodendri), Yi Yi Ren(Semen Coicis), Dang Gui (Radix Angelicae Sinensis), Tao Ren(Semen Persicae), Hong Hua (Flos Carthami), Chi Shao (Radix Paeoniae Rubra), Dan Shen (Radix Salviae Miltiorrhizae), Shui Zhi(Hirudo), Jiang Can(Bambyx Batryticatus), Jin Yin Hua (Flos Lonicerae), Pu Gong Ying (Herba Taraxaci), Lian Qiao(Fructus Forsythiae), Bai Lian(Radix Ampelopsis), Chan Yi (Periostracum Cicadae), Ye Ju Hua (Flos Achyranthemi Indici), Niu Xi(Radix Achyranthis Bidentatae), etc.

7. 5. 4 Case Study

Case 1.

Chen was a 58 years old male cadre in a candy factory, who had polydipsia and blurred vision for two years and diabrosis of the left big toe for half a month. He was admitted on March 16, 1991 after a disgnosis of diabetic foot was made.

The patient was found to have diabetes three years ago. Since then, he had been treated with a number of hypoglycemic agents, which were not so effective. When he was admitted, he had polydipsia, polyphagia, loss of weight(his weight was reduced by 10 kg within the past two years), blurred vision, cold feet with aversion to cold, pain and a dark purple colour which was more obvious and became piebald shape when the legs were falling. The dorsum and top of his left big toe were diabrotic with exudates, his tongue was dark red with thin and whitish coating, and his pulse was thready and uneven. Laboratory test revealed that the blood sugar was 14. 5 mmol/L and the urine glucose was(+ + + +). Test of ketone in the urine was positive but proteinuria was not detected. The serum total cholesterol was 8 mmol/L, triglyceride was 4mmol/L and the blood pressure was 24/14. 7 kPa. Then he was diagnosed as having diabetes, type II, which was complicated by gangrene and hyperlipemia in the view of Western medicine and qi deficency, blood stasis, obstruction of vessles and accumulation of toxic heat in the interior in the view of TCM.

Therapeutic method: Supplementing qi, activating blood flow, warming up channels and removing obstruction of the collaterals, assisted by clearing away heat and removing toxic materials.

Prescription:

① Glybenzcyclamide, to be taken 2. 5mg each time, three times daily.

② Huang Qi (Radix Astragali seu Hedysari) 30g, Dan Shen (Radix Salviae Miltiorrhizae) 30g, Ji Xue Teng(Caulis Spatholobi) 30g, Jin Yin Hua (Flos Lonicerae) 30g, Pu Gong Ying (Herba Taraxaci) 30g, Gui Zhi (Ramulus Cinnamomi) 12g, Lu Lu Tong (Fructus Liquidambaris) 12g, Hang Shao (Chinese Herbaceous Peony) 20g, Chuan Xiong (Rhizoma Ligustici Chuanxiong) 20g, Mu Gua (Fructus Chaenomelis) 15g, Ge Gen (Radix Puerariae) 15g, Tu Fu Ling (Rhizoma Smilacis Glabrae) 15g, Hong Hua (Flos

Carthami) 10g, and Gan Cao(Radix Glyyrrhizae) 6g, to be decocted in water for oral use.

③ Leech tincture, to be smeared on the affected part three to four times daily.

The ulcer was healed about 20 days later with the administration of the above drugs with modifications. Then Huoxue Zhitong San (Powder for Activating Blood and Relieving Pain) was also prescribed to fumigate and wash the affected area, one dose daily. Fifty-three days later, the color and temperature of the feet restored to normal and the pain disappeared. His blood sugar was 9 mmol/L and the urine glucose was ++ to +∼. Then he was discharged with a pleasure. After that he was instructed to continue the treatment for diabetes.

Case 2.

Diao was a 63 year-old female retired worker who was found to have diabetes five years ago. In the past two years, she developed coldness of the feet with aversion to cold, and in the recent one month, the symptoms of polydipsia and lassitude became worse. Besides, blisters occurred on the toes without any reason, followed by diabrosis and and discharge of pus half a month ago. She had been treated with glybenzcyclamide since she had diabetes, and she had no history of drinking and smoking and family history of diabetes. She was admitted after being diganosed as having diabetic gangrene in the out-patient department on Janurary 22, 1991.

When she was admitted, she had polydipsia and polyuria, diabrosis with discharge of pus on her right big toe and the bottom of metatarsus with unbearable pain, and dry stool. Physical examination: senile female with consciousness, suffering expression, dark red tongue with dry, thin and whitish coating, wiry and thready pulse. Body temperature: 36℃; pulse: 86 beats per minute; respiration: 18 periods per minute, and the blood pressure: 21/9 kPa. ECG: approximately normal; the lung and the heart(−). The skin

186

of the feet was dark purple with a lowered temperature and a cold feeling, diabrosis and discharge of pus on the big toes and the bottom of the metatarsus with an elevated skin temperature in the local area, and the arteriopalmus beats were reduced. Laboratory tests: blood sugar, 12. 8 mmol/L, cholesterol, 6. 2 mmol/L, triglyceride, 1. 5 mmol/L, quanlitative test for glucose in the urine, $++++$, qualitative test for the ketone in the urine, $\pm$, and the qualitative test for protein in the urine, $+$.

Diagnosis: Diabetic gangrene of feet in the view of Western medicine, qi deficiency, blood stasis and accumulation of toxic heat in the interior in the view of TCM.

Therapeutic method: Supplementing qi, activating blood flow, removing blood stasis and clearing away heat and removing toxic materials.

Prescriptions:

①Combined Neituo Shengji San (Powder for Replenishing Qi and Blood to Promote Tissue Regeneration) and Simiao Yongan Tang (Decoction of Four Wonderful Drugs for Detoxicating and Activating Blood Circulation) with modifications:

Huang Qi (Radix Astragali seu Hedysari) 30g, Dang Shen (Radix Codonopsis Pilosulae) 15g, Dang Gui (Radix Angelicae Sinensis) 15g, Bai Zhi (Radix Dahuricae) 10g, Chuan Xiong (Rhizoma Ligustri Chuanxiong) 15g, Dan Shen (Radix Salviae Miltiorrhizae) 30g, Cang Zhu (RHizoma Atractylodis) 12g, Niu Xi (Radix Achyranthis Bidentatae) 15g, Huang Bai (Cortex Phellodendri) 9g, Tu Fu Ling (Rhizoma Smilacis Glabrae) 15g, Jin Yin Hua (Flos Lonicerae) 30g, Zao Jiao Ci (Spina Gleditsiae) 15g, to be decocted in water for oral use, one dose daily.

② Leech tincture, to be applied to the affected part after the wound is cleaned.

With modifications in accordance with the changes of the disease, 30 doses or more of the Chinese herbal medicine formula were administered, as a result, discharge of pus disappeared. More two months later, the wound healed, the blood sugar was controlled around 7 mmol/L. Then the decoction of formula was stopped, and the proprietaries Xiaoke Ping and Xiaoke Wan were prescribed to control the blood sugar in succession. When she was discharged, she was prescribed the following prescription:

Huang Qi(Radix Astragali seu Hedysari) 30g, Gui Zhi(Ramulus Cinnamomi) 10g, Hang Shao(Chinese Herbaceous Peony) 15g, Dan Shen (Radix Salviae Miltiorrhizae) 30g, Chuan Xiong (Rhizoma Ligustici Chuanxiong) 15g, Chi Shao(Radix Paeoniae Rubra) 15g, Hong Hua(Flos Carthami) 10g, and Gan Cao(Radix Glycyrrhizae) 6g, to be decocted in water for oral administration.

She was also advised to take the above prescription constantly to improve the blood circulation in the local area and do more exercise of the limbs to prevent diabrosis and infection of the feet.

7. 6 Diabetes complicated by impotence

This is a syndrome involving the urogenital nerves in diabetes and is a commonly seen complication in male diabetics, which accounts for $40-50\%$ of the complications of diabetes in male according to the reports from other countries, and 21% according to the reports from China. Disturbance of the sacral vegetative nerve is concerned in the occurrence of the disease.

The disease has a slow onset, manifested as inability of the penis to erect but still with sexuality at the early stage, and occurrence of the other symptoms of disturbance of the vegetative nerve at the later stage. Usually it takes six to twenty-four months for the mild impotence to develop to the complete one and sterility often presents as a consequence in the young males.

Diabetic impotence should be distinguished from the impotence secondary to psychogenic neurasthenia. The latter occurs mainly in the young and has an acute onset. It is a paroxysmal condition related to

188

emotional states, usually caused by vexation due to errorneous selection of wife or emotional stress during the sexual activities, and may be accompanied with nocturnal emission. But the patients still have sexuality. Impotence secondary to diabetes usually presents progressive aggravation of the symptoms due to loss of control of the blood glucose and will eventually lead to loss of sexuality, but no nocturnal emission is accompanied.

In TCM, this disease was named Yin Wei(Flaccidity of the Penis) in chapter of Varities of Visceral Disease of the book *Miraculous Pivot*, or Yinqi Buyong(Debility of the penis) in the chapter of On Channels and Tendons of the same book. Its pathogenesis lies in that prolonged diabetes impairs the spleen and the kidney, causing deficiency of qi and blood and consumption of the essence, or that decline of fire of mingmen fails to activate the erection of the penis. Through ages, most doctors believed that the diseases involves mainly the Liver Meridian, the Kidney Meridian and the Yangming Meridian (the Stomach Meridian). Therefore, TCM treatment on the disease should be performed according to the results of syndrome identification and the clinical manifestations of the disease while the blood sugar and other conditions of diabetes are controlled.

7. 6. 1 Type of decline of mingmen-fire

Main Manifestations: Impotence, pale complexion, dizziness, vertigo, listlessness, soreness and weakness of the loins and knees, absence of polydipsia, polyphagia and polyuria, elevation of the blood sugar and urine glucose, pale tongue with whitish coating, deep and thready pulse.

Therapeutic method: Tonifying the kidney and warming up yang.

Prescription: Zanyu Dan (Bolus for Nourishing the Kidney-essence, from *Jingyue's Complete Medical Books*), ingredients of which are:

Shu Di(Radix Rehmanniae Praeparata) 12g, Dang Gui(Radix Angelicae Sinensis) 12g, Ba Ji Tian(Radix Morindae Officinalis) 12g,

Rou Cong Rong (Herba Cistanchis) 12g, Gou Qi Zi (Fructus Lycii) 12g, Xian Ling Pi (Herba Epimedii) 12g, Shan Yu Rou (Fructus Corni) 12g, Du Zhong (Cortex Eucommiae) 10g, Bai Zhu (Rhizoma Atractylodis Macrocephalae) 10g, Xian Mao (Rhizoma Curculignis) 10g, She Chuang Zi (Fructus Cnidii) 9g, Rou Gui (Cortex Cinnamomi) 9g, Jiu Zi (Semen Allii Tuberosi) 15g, Fu Zi (Radix Aconiti) 6g, and Ren Shen (Radix Ginseng) 6g, to be decocted in water for oral dose.

For cases with spermatorrhea and premature ejaculation, Wuzi Yanzong Wan (Bolus of Five Semens for Treating Sterility, from *Danxi's Experiential Therapy*) with modifications may be adopted, ingredients of which are:

Gou Qi Zi (Fructus Lycii) 15g, Fu Pen Zi (Fruuctus Rubi) 15g, Tu Si Zi (Semen Cuscutae) 20g, Wu Wei Zi (Fructus Schisandrae) 10g, Che Qian Zi (Semen Plantaginis) 30g, Shan Yao (Rhizoma Dioscoreae) 15g, Shan Yu Rou (Fructus Corni) 15g, Shu Di (Radix Rehmanniae Praeparata) 15g, Sheng Di (Radix Rehmanniae) 15g, Qian Shi (Semen Euryales) 15g, Xian Ling Pi (Herba Epimedii) 12g, Jin Ying Zi (Fructus Rosae Laevigatae) 20g, Gan Cao (Radix Glycyrrhizae) 6g, to be decocted in water for oral use.

By comparison, Zanyu Dan has a better effect on warming the kidney, while Wuzi Yanzong Wan has a powerful effect on consolidating essence. In the treatment of impotence, both warming up yang ad nourishing essence should be adopted simultaneously so that the kidney yin and the kidney yang can promote each other. Usually, drugs sweet in taste and warm in nature, those salty in taste and warm in nature, or those with nourishing effects are what should be employed, while those bitter in taste and cold in nature with the action of purgation, those with the action of inducing diuresis, those bitter in taste and dry in nature, those with drastic qi stagnation-relieving effect, or those with dispersing effect, should not be used indiscriminately.

7.6.2 Type of deficiency of both the heart and the spleen and deficiency of both qi and blood

Main manifestations: Impotence, listlessness, insomnia, lustreless complexion, pale tongue with thin and greasy tongue coating, and thready pulse.

Therapeutic method: Tonifying the heart and the spleen, regulating qi and blood.

Prescription: Gui Pi Tang (Decoction for Invigorating the Spleen and Nourishing the Heart, from *Prescriptions for Benevolence*) with modification, ingredients of which are:

Huang Qi (Radix Astragali seu Hedysari) 30g, Dang Shen (Radix Codonopsis Pilosulae) 20g, Fu Ling (Poria), Mai Dong (Radix Ophiopogonis) 12g, Long Yan Rou (Arillus Longan) 20g, Dang Gui (Radix Angelicae Sinensis) 15g, Gou Qi Zi (Fructus Lycii) 15g, Mu Xiang (Radix Aucklandiae) 9g, Yuan Zhi (Radix Polygalae Praeparata) 9g, Suan Zao Ren (Fructus Ziziphi Spinosae) 30g, Wu Wei Zi (Fructus Shisandrae) 10g, Gan Cao (Radix Glycyrrhizae) 6g, to be decocted in water for oral dose.

For the impotence due to anxiety, terror and fright impairing the spleen and the kidney, Qifu Yin (Drink of Seven Happiness, from *Jingyue's Complete Medical Books*) with modifiication should be adopted, which consists of:

Ren Shen (Radix Ginseng) 9g, Bai Zhu (Rhizoma Atractylodis Macrocephalae) 15g, Shu Di (Radix Rehmanniae Praeparata) 15g, Dang Gui (Radix Angelicae Sinensis) 15g, Shan Yao (Rhizoma Dioscoreae) 15g, Shan Yu Rou (Fructus Corni) 15g, Zhi Yuan Zhi (Radix Polygalae Praeparata) 10g, Suan Zao Ren (Fructus Ziziphi Spinosae) 30g, Xian Ling Pi (Herba Epimedii) 12g, Zhi Gan Cao (Radix Glycyrrhizae Praeparata) 6g, to be decocted in water for oral dose.

7.6.3 Type of fright impairing the kidney

Main manifestations: Impotence, mental depression, timidness, inclination to lie flat, palpitation, insomnia, thin and greasy tongue coating, or bluish tongue, wiry and thready pulse.

Therapeutic method: Benefiting the kidney and calming the mind.

Prescription: Da Buyuan Jian (Major Decoction for Tonifying the Primordial Qi, from *Jingyue's Complete Medical Books*) with modification, ingredients of which are:

Ren Shen (Radix Ginseng) 9g, Chao Shan Yao (Rhizoma Dioscoreae, stir-fried) 15g, Shu Di Huang (Radix Rehmanniae Praeparata) 15g, Dang Gui (Radix Angelicae Sinensis) 15g, Shan Yu Rou (Fructus Corni) 15g, Du Zhong (Cortex Eucommiae) 10g, Gou Qi Zi (Fructus Lycii) 10g, Xian Ling Pi (Herba Epidemii) 12g, Mai Dong (Radix Ophiopogonis) 12g, Wu Wei Zi (Fructus Schisandrae) 9g, Zhi Yuan Zhi (Radix Polygalae Praeparata) 9g, Chao Suan Zao Ren (Fructus Ziziphi Spinosae, stir-fried) 30g, Gan Cao (Radix Glycyrrhizae) 6g, to be decocted in water for oral dose.

This type is mostly seen in psychogenic impotence, usually caused by sudden fright impairing the kidney-yang and is marked by sudden occurrence of impotence. Therefore, the treatment should be aimed at tonifying the kidney. Impotence in the newly-married with a strong constitution is mostly of this type, which should be treated by relieving the mental depression in combination.

7. 6. 4 Type of downward flow of dampness-heat

Main manifestations: Impotence, scanty and dark urine, soreness and heaviness of the lower limbs, or complicated by nocturnal emission, yellow and greasy tongue coating, soft, slippery and rapid pulse.

Impotence of this type is caused by the dampness-heat flowing downward leading to relaxation of tendons.

Therapeutic method: Clearing away heat and removing dampness.

Prescription: Zhibai Dihuang Tang (Rehmannia Root Decoction with Anemarrhena Rhizome and Phellodendron Bark, from *The Golden Mirror of Medicine*) with modification, ingredients of which are:

Zhi Mu (Rhizoma Anemarrhenae) 10g, Huang Bai (Cortex Phellodendri) 10g, Shu Di(Radix Paeoniae Praeparata) 12g, Shan Yu Rou(Fructus Corni) 12g, Shan Yao(Rhizoma Dioscorae) 15g, Fu Ling(Poria) 15g, Dan Pi(Cortex Moutan Radicis) 15g, Cang Zhu (Rhizoma Atractylodis) 20g, Niu Xi(Radix Achyranthis Bidentatae) 15g, to be decocted in water for oral use.

For cases with prostatitis, the drugs of Western medicine should be applied in combination to control the inflammation, or Jin Yin Hua (Flos Lonicerae) 30g, Pu Gong Ying(herba Taraxaci) 20g, Bai Mao Gen(Rhizoma Imperatae) 30g, etc., should be added to the above prescription.

Impotence of dampness-heat type is a rare condition, but the yellow and greasy tongue coating occurring in this type is rather difficult to treat. As the patients who are eager to be cured may take tonic drugs, which would make the condition more complicated and severe, the patients' condition must be carefully examined in the clinic. For those with dampness-heat, clearing away heat and removing dampness must be employed first in the treatment.

In addition, for cases with depletion of the essence-qi, impotence in males, or asexuality in females, the following proved formula may be administered in combination:

Ge Jie(Gecko) one pair, Ren Shen(Radix Ginseng) 10g, Hai Ma (Hippocampus) 10g, Gou Qi Zi(Fructus Lycii) 30g, Xian Ling Pi (Herba Epidemii) 20g, Ba Ji Tian(Radix Morindae) 20g, Shan Yao (Rhizoma Dioscoreae) 20g, Dang Gui (Radix Angelicae Sinensis) 20g, ox penis(two pieces), and sheep testicle(two pieces).

The above drugs are ground into powder after being baked, then put into capsules to be taken 4 pills each time, three times daily. Effectiveness can be expected after one or two doses are administered.

In brief, about 70—80% of the male patients with diabetes will develop impotence, which is usually more severe than that caused by other conditions. It occurs slowly, but it may develop into organic impotence in a chronic case and is difficult to cure. Therefore, positive treatment should be taken to control the blood glucose, or to control the infection first in the case of urinary infection or prostatitis. Moreover, drugs promoting blood flow and removing blood stasis should be added deliberately in the treatment, so as to obtain even better therapeutic effects. Be sure not to treat the impotence simply without treating the other complicated diseases.

7. 6. 5 Case Study

Case 1.

Zuo was a 45 years old male who began to have polydipsia, polyphagia and polyuria in March of 1978. He was found to have a fasting blood glucose of 11. 1mmol/L and a urine glucose of +++ in a hospital in New York. He had had diet-control therapy since then, but had never received medication treatment. He developed impotence in 1982, which still existed. Recently, his condition was gradually aggravated and he was in a mental depression.

On examination, he had dry mouth, which was milder in the daytime and severe at night, emaciation, lassitude, distension of the hypochondrium, impotence, lowered temperature of the limbs, dark tongue with teethmarks on the margin and thin coating, and wiry pulse. His fasting urine glucose was found to be +++. Then he was diagnosed as having deficiency of yang-qi complicated by stagnation of qi.

Therapeutic method: Warming the kidney, strengthening yang, supplementing qi and relieving the liver depression.

Prescription: Huang Qi(Radix Astragali seu Hedysari) 50g, Wu Wei Zi(Fructus Schisandrae) 12g, Shan Yu Rou(Fructus Corni) 20g, Fu Zi(Radix Aconiti) 9g, Sang Piao Xiao(Ootheca Mantidis) 12g, Sheng Long Gu(Os Draconis) 30g, Sheng Mu Li(Concha Ostreae) 30g, Chai Hu(Radix Bupleuri, stir-fried with vinegar) 9g, Bai Shao(Radix Paeoniae Alba, stir-fried with vinegar) 9g, Bai Ji Li(Fructus Tribuli) 9g, to be decocted in water for oral dose.

After fifteen doses were administered, he made his second visit.

194

Dry mouth and distension of the hypochondrium disappeared and the other symptoms were relieved. The blood sugar was normal. His pulse was wiry and his tongue was dark and slightly tender. These showed that satisfactory effect had been obtained. Then the original formula was continued with proper midification:

Huang Qi (Radix Astragali seu Hedysari) 50g, Shan Yu Rou (Fructus Corni) 20g, Wu Wei Zi (fruuctus Schisandrae) 12g, Sang Piao Xiao (Ootheca Mantidis) 9g, Sheng Long Gu (os Draconis) 12g, Sheng Mu Li (Concha Ostreae) 12g, Ji Nei Jin (Endothelium Corneum Gigeriae Galli, to be taken after being ground into powder) 10g, Fu Zi (Radix Aconiti) 9g, Bai Ji Li (Fructus Tribuli) 9g, Rou Cong Rong (Herba Cistanchis) 15g, to be decocted in water for oral dose.

On the New Year of 1984, he told the doctor by letter that his impotence as well as other symptoms had been cured after 20 doses of the formula were administered, his fasting blood sugar was 5.5 mmol/L and the urine glucose was negative through several tests. Then he was told to take Jinkui Shengqi Wan (Bolus for Tonifying the Kidney-Qi from *Synopsis of Prescriptions of the Gold Chamber*) for one month to fortify the therapeutic effects. (From *Diagnosis and Treatment of Diabetes in TCM*, Written by Li Liang)

Notes: Diabetes complicated by impotence is a commonly seen disease in the clinic. This case arises from weakness of yang-qi and decline of mingmen-fire due to over anxiety and mental depression, excessive sexual activities and the original diabetes. An ancient doctor said: " when a disease occurs, treat it with corresponding drugs", so the therapeutic principle of tonifying the kidney, invigorating yang and relieving the liver depression were employed in the treatment of this case.

Case 2.

Zhang was a 38 years old female cardre in the rural area who paid her first visit on April 20, 1990. She had been ill with diabetes for 5 years and the blood sugar was 12. 0 mmol/L, the urine glucose was +++++ and the cholesterol was normal when the disease was first found. She had been treated with glybenzcyclamide which occasionally reduced the blood sugar to be 7 mmol/L. She had not obvious polydipsia, polyphagia and polyuria. She was married at 23 years old and gave birth to a healthy boby at 25 years old. She had two abortions and her menstrual circle was normal, but the mense was less. No gynecological diseases were found and her husband was healthy. In the past two years, she began to have progressive asexuality and lost orgasm, which made her fail to have sexual intercourse. She was ashamed to tell her condition even to the doctor, so she and her family suffered a lot from this.

Trusting the doctor, she told the doctor all the above when she came for her visit. According to her condition, TCM diagnosis of syndrome was made, which showed that her condition was caused by deficiency of the kidney-yang and decline of the mingmen-fire. So the treatment was aimed at tonifying the kidney, warming up yang and invigorating the kidney-qi. Drugs prescribed were: Ge Jie (Gecko) two pieces, Ren Shen (Radix Ginseng) 15g, Hai Ma (Hippocampus) 15g, Gou Qi Zi (Fructus Lycii) 30g, Xian Ling Pi (Herba Epimedii) 15g, Xian Mao (Rhizoma Curculiginis) 10g, Ba Ji Tian (Radix Morindae Officinalis) 10g, Shan Yao (Rhizoma Dioscoreae) 15g, Dang Gui (Radix Angelicae Sinensis) 12g, Shan Yu Rou (Fructus Corni) 20g, Niu Bian (Ox Penis) one piece, to be ground into fine powder after being ground and taken in the form of capsule, 4 pills each time, three times daily. She was also instructed to take one sea cucumber each day. She experienced improvement after one dose of the formula was administered. And her sexual function restored to normal after 3 more doses were continued. But she was advised to continue the treatment for her diabetes.

196

Chapter 8   Diet Therapy
and Medicated Diet

Diet therapy is an essential therapy for diabetes and the prerequisite of all the other therapies. No matter which type of the diabetes it is, how serious it is and whether there is complication, the patient must strictly carry on and persist long term diet control. However, diet therapy is often neglected by both doctors and patients clinically. Some patients do know it but never follow it. In mild cases, diet therapy alone may control the disease. And in severe cases or those with insulin therapy, a well controlled diet in combination with other therapies will bring about satisfactory therapeutic effects.

To take diatetic therapy, patients should, first of all, realize the importance of this therapy and master its laws and principle. Besides, they must keep on it for a long time. Medicated diet and diet therapy in TCM can promote the production of body fluid, relieve hunger and improve the patients' constitutions, so they can control the disease.

8. 1 Single drug or food

1) Shan Yao(Rhizoma Dioscoreae): It has certain effect on the Xiaoke Syndrome(mild or moderate diabetes). It may be taken as food or the decoction of 250 g of it can be taken as tea for long use.

2) Cushaw powder(Pulvis Cucurbitae Moschatae): it is administered 30g each day for one to three months. The longer the time is, the better the therapeutic effects will be.

3) Huang Qi(Radix Astragali seu Hedysari) ; It is recorded in *Qian Jin Fang* (*Presciptions Worthing One Thousand Golds*) that Huang Qi is effective for Xiaoke syndrome. 30—50g of Huang Qi are to be stewed

with old hen to be taken orally.

4) Gou Qi Zi(Fructus Lycii): It is often used as a supplement of dishes, such as wolfberry fruit broth and broth of wolfberry fruit and pig's liver, among the Chinese people. As it is bright red in colour, it can make the food more beutiful. 6-12g are to be taken for diabetics.

5) Tian Hua Fen(Radix Trichosanthis): Take 3—12g of the fresh drug or the decoction of the drug for diabetes of type II marked by severe thirst with excessive drinks, dry mouth and tongue and polyphagia.

6) Dong Gua(Benincasae): Drinking a lot of the juice made from pounded fresh wax courd can be used to treat severe thirst with desire for drinks caused by diabetes.

7) Cong(Chinese onion): Modern medicine has proved that this drug has a better effect of lowering the blood glucose. It can be used long as food or a drug for diabetes.

8) Radish: The juice of the pounded radish taken orally is highly effective for diabetes. According to Western medicine, diabetes often develops specific abnormality of the small and minor vessels and obstruction of the pancreatic vessels. Radish has the function of removing blood stasis,so it can relieve the above conditions and restore the normal secretion of the pancreas.

9) Meat of the soft shelled-turtle: Remove the visera of a soft shelled turtle, clean it with water and then decoct it in water with some salt. When it is ready, eat the meat and drink the soap. This has an obvious effect of lowering the blood glucose and is especially suitale for diabetics with severe emaciation.

10) Ricefield eel: diabetics with type II may take the fresh of the eel by cooking it into dishes, 60-90g each day. Usually the blood sugar and the urine glucose will decrease in three to four weeks.

11) Mushroom: Frequent intake of mushroom has an obvious effect on the prevention of the complications of diabetes.

8. 2 Commonly used formulas

1) Mung been 200g, pear 2 pieces, green radish 250g, to be taken after being decocted and well done together.

2) Rice crust 200g, lotus seed 100g, to be taken after being decocted together.

3) Spinach root 200g, American fresh ginger 50g, to be decocted together to produce juice for oral use.

4) Gruel of radish: Have 250g of fresh radish boiled until it is well done. Then get the juice of it and then mix it with 100g of polished round-grained rice to make gruel for oral use.

5) Soup of pork tripe: Fat pork tripe (washed clean) 1 piece, green Chinese onion a handful, fermented sojae been (wrapped with silk floss) 5 small boxes. Stew the pork tripe first until it is thoroughly done, then add the other two ingredients. Cut the pork tripe into slices to be taken when hungery and drink the soup when thirst.

6) Gruel of wolfberry fruit: wolfberry fruit 15—20g, polished glutinous rice 50g, to be taken after being decocted together.

7) Gruel of Di Huang(Radix Rehmannia): Di Huang(fresh Radix Rehmanniae) 150g, polished glutinous rice 50g. Wrap the pounded Di Huang with a cloth and then squeez it to get juice. Add the juice to the soup made from the polished glutinous rice and 500ml of water to decoct them together with soft fire for some minutes. Take the gruel two to three times a day while it is warm.

8) Fragrant solomonseal rhizome 15—20g, or the fresh 30—60g, polished round-grained rice 100g. Wash the fresh fragrant solomonseal rhizome clean and take its roots off, then cut it into small pieces to get juice and discard the dregs. Add the polished round-grained rice and the water as appropriate to make thin gruel to be taken in the morning and evening.

9) Gruel of Trichosanthes root: Hua Fen(Radix Trichosanthes) 15g, polished round-grained rice 100g, to be made into gruel and tak-

en twice daily.

10) Gruel of spinach root: Fresh spinach root 250g, chicken's gizzard-skin 10g, rice as appropriate. First wash the spinach root clean and cut it into pieces. Put the chisken's gizzard-skin and water as appropriate to it and decoct them together for half a hour, then add in the washed rice to make gruel.

Take the gruel several times a day.

11) Proper amount of han Yao (Rhizoma Diocoreae) and sheep tripe: Boil the sheep strip in water until it is well-done, then add han Yao to be decocted together until they are both well-done, then add some salt to the decoction. Take them at an empty stomach, once daily.

12) Soup of pork bones and Tu Fu Ling (Rhizoma Smilacis Glabrae): Pork backbone, 500g, and Tu Fu Ling 50-100g. Stew the pork backbone in proper amount of water to be as much as 3 bowels can contain, remove the bones and the suspensious oil. Then decoct the left with Tu Fu Ling to be as much as two bowles can contain. Take the decoction fully by two times within a day.

13) Thick soup of pork spine: Pork spine 1 piece, Chinese date 150g, Lian Zi (Semen Nelumbinis, the core removed) 100g, Mu Xiang (Radix Aucklandiae) 3g, and Gan Cao (Radix Glycyrrhizae) 10g. Clean the pork bones with water and cut it into pieces, and wrap Mu Xiang and Gan Cao with a piece of gauze. Put all the ingredients in a pot to be stewed with proper amount of water over four hours under soft fire. Take it by meals, drinking the soup and eating the meat, dates and lotus seed.

14) Steamed Crucian carp stuffed with tea: Crucian carp 500g and green tea proper amount. Put the green tea into the belly of the crucian carp whose gill, intestines and visera have been removed, to be stewed in a pot and taken the stewed fish once daily.

15) Drink of Bai Guo (Semen Ginkgo, shelled) and Yi Mi (Semen Coicis): Bai Guo 8—10 pieces, Yi Mi 100g, to be decocted in water

as appropriate to be taken twice daily.

16) Duck stuffed with Qian Shi(Semen Euryales): One old duck and 200g Qian Shi. Stuff Qian Shi into the duck abdomen and stew them together in an earthware with clear water for some two hours with soft fire, then add some salt to make taste and take them by oral.

17) Duck stuffed with Dong Chong Xia Cao(Cordyceps): One old male duck and 15g of Dong Chong Xia Cao. Remove the hair and viscera of the duck, put Dong Chong Xia Cao and some water into the abdomen, to be baked in a small earthpot. When it is well-done, take it as meal. (As a dish, it is used as tonic in China. Female duck can also be used if there is no the male.)

18) Tortoise soup with Yu Mi Xu(Corn stigma): Yu Mi Xu 60—120g(or the dry stigma, 30—60g) and one or two tortoise. Scald tortoise with boling water to make it urinates thoroughly, remove its viscera, head and paws and wash it clean. Then put its meat with corn stigma in a earthware to be stewed with some clear water in soft fire. Eat the meat and drink the soup.

19) Tea gruel: Black tea 2g, polished glutinous rice 50—100g, water 600—800ml. When the water is boiling, add the polished glutinous rice, and add the tea when the rice is well-done. The gruel is taken warm, twice a day and for one day's use.

20) Tea with luffa: Tea 5g and luffa 200g. Cut the cleaned luffa in to the slices of 0.66cm in thickness, then decoct it in salty water until it is thoroughly done. Add the water infused with the tea to the decoction to be taken twice a day.

21) Crucian carp stuffed with tea: Green tea 10g and living crucian carp 500g. Remove the viscera of the fish and wash it clean, then stuff the tea into the abdomen of the fish to be placed on a plate. Steam them together without salt and then take the fish once daily.

22) Decoction of tea and ginger: Green tea 6g, fresh ginger 2

slices, and salt 4. 5g, to be decocted together to get 500ml of decoction and taken several times.

23) Won ton with rabbit meat: Rabbit meat 100g, flour 250g, one egg, and appropriate amount of bean flour, salt, gourmet powder and Chinese onion. Chop the meat into the ground meat, put into bean flour, salt, gourment powder and Chinese onion and stir them together thoroughly. Then make dumpling wrappers with the prepared meat with the flour in a routine way, to be boiled in water and taken as meal.

Chapter 9 Other Therapies of
Traditional Chinese Medicine

9. 1 Qigong Therapy

As early as in the Jin Dynasty, application of qigong therapy to diabetes had been recorded in *Zhu Bing Yuan Hou Lun* (*Treatise on Causes and Syndromes of Diseases*), the earliest monograph on syndromes of TCM. In recent years, many studies showing that qigong is very effective for the disease were also reported. According to the test made by the Physiology Section of the First Shanghai Medical University, qigong exercise can quickly decrease the blood sugar concentration and enhance the glycometabolism.

9. 1. 1 Methods to exercise qigong therapy

Method One: Take a lying or sitting position, relax the whole body with the eyes slightly closed and the palate supported by the tongue, then breathe by inhaling, exhaling and pause alternatively with the mind concentrated on dantian and say "Zi Ji Jing "(calming myself) to oneself by heart. That is, say "Zi" when inhaling, "Ji" when exhaling and "Jing" before next circle of breath. The saliva increased can be sent down to dantian freely under the guidance of one's mind.

This method is to be performed 3 times and 3 — 5 hours a day in the morning, noon and evening respectively.

Method Two: Stand with the body relaxed and the mind calmed, close the eyes slightly and promt the palate with the tongue (this can increase the secretion of the saliva to relieve thirst in a short time). The abdomen should be expanded as much as possible during inspiration until its maximum, and depressed gradually during respiration to be the nearest to the spinal column. The respiration should be even, long and deep so that the amplitude of the diaphragm movement is increased and the stomach as well as the pancreas, due to the movement of the pulmonary muscles, are massaged and the amount of pancreas cells increased. After 50 times, one should concentrate his or her mind on the epigastric region to become calm, which can help to regulate the blood sugar concentration. Improvement of glucose tolerance during qigong exercise may be a result of the accelerated hyposthesis and reduced decomposition of the hepatic glycogen.

This method is performed three times a day in the morning, noon and evening, 30 to 60 minutes each time.

Method Three: Lying flat with the cloth taken off, calm one's mind and get rid of distractions, support the upper palate with the tongue, relax the whole body, and stretch out the loins and legs. Take an abdominal respiration and strive for expending the lower abdomen. Breath in 5 times first, then stop breathing in and begin to breath out while the mind induces the decrease of blood sugar.

This method is performed three times a day in the morning, noon and evening, 30 to 60 minutes each time.

Method Four: Sit on the bed or a stool with the cloth untied. The feet is firstly placed naturally by curving one leg or crossing the both. Then the two hands are overlaped on the legs just anterior to the lower abodmen by putting the palm of the right hand over the left. Then move the body right and left for 7 to 8 times to make the body upstand and the nose at the same horizonal line with the umbilicus. Be sure not to bend or bend back. Open the mouth to give off the turbid qi in the abdomen, then, with the tongue supporting the upper palate, breath in the fresh air through the nose and mouth 3 to 7 times, after which the mouth is shut. The lips and the teeth then are kept close and the upper palate is still supported by the tongue. Continue the posture with the eyes slighly closed for some time. During doing so, if the body is not upright, correct it slowly at times. Af-

204

ter that, open the mouth to breath out several ten times to disperse the heat in the body, and shake the whole body gently, then the scapula and the head and neck, and then relax the two hands. The two thumbs should then rub each other to produce heat and then be moved to rub the eyelids, the nose and its two sides. Rub the palms again to produce heat and to rub the auricles and the whole body in the orders of the head, chest, abdomen, back, arms, feet, legs and the soles. Then, the respiration is regulated to be extremely slow, mild and even and the mind is concentrated on dantian for 10 to 30 minutes.

The best time is from one hour before to one hour after the midnight, or from three to five o'clock in the morning in a silent room, 3 to 4 times a day and 30 to 40 minutes each time. The effect of this method usually occurs in one month or so, and the symptoms can be controlled within 3 to 4 months. After the relief of the symptoms, the method should be continued, 20 to 30 minutes each time, once daily, to fortify the therapeutic effect.

Method Five: Take a sitting or standing position and get rid of distractions. Concentrate on the tip of nose a while then close the eyes to see inward the epigastric region. Listen carefully the expiration to avoid coarse breath and induce the mind to the epigastric region, and keep the mind free during inhalation. The genuine qi will gather in the epigastric region after repeated the method. It is required to do the exercise three times a day in the morning, noon and evening, 20 minutes each time. The above is the first stage of the exercise.

When one can feel hot in his epigastric region as long as exhaling, the hot feeling should be induced to go down to the dantian gradually. This is to be done 3 times a day, 25 to 30 minutes each time.

When a strong feeling in dantian is felt, the respiration should be retained in dantian. Do this 3 times a day, 30 minutes or more each time. This is the third stage.

40 days or so after the third stage, the genuine qi will fill the dan-

tian to a certain degree. That means, the genuine qi in dantian is sufficient enough to go upward along the spinal column. If it stops somewhere, do not induce it upward with the mind. It will gradually go upward after the further accumulation of the genuine qi. If it stops in the occipital region one will be able to see inward the summit of the head, and the exercising times in a day should be increased and the time of each exercise should be from 40 to 60 minutes. This is the fourth stage.

The last stage is to concentrate the mind on the dantian or the summit of the head if a motion is felt in Baihui(DU 20) or other regions, 3 times a day, 60 minutes or more each time.

This method must be exercised step by step. The practitioner should avoid anxiety and strive for progress by persistent exercise to reach the goal. After Du Meridian begins to circulate, the disease will be relieved markedly and the sugar in the blood and urine became normal gradually. Besides one will also feel vigorous and comfortable.

Notes:

(1) Qigong therapy can be applied at the same time with the drug therapy to diabetic patients, it can strengthen the effect of the drugs. When the effect comes to emerge, the drugs can be gradually stopped and qigong therapy should be the main therapy. This can not only fortify the therapeutic effect but also prevent its recurrence.

(2) The qigong exercise should be continued when the diabetes is controlled, but the times and the time for one exercise should be reduced. This can fortify the therapeutic effect, prevent its reattack, make the body stronger and prolong life.

(3) Combined use of qigong therapy and massage of Zusanli(ST 30) and Yongquan(KI 1) may enhance the effect. The details are as follows:

① Rubbing Zusanli(ST 30), the points located 3 cun below the knees on the bilateral sides, with the bellies of the two thumbs at the

206

same time 50 times. This can regulate the function of the gastrointestinal tract, induce the heart fire to go down and the kidney fire to go up.

② Massage on Yongquan (KI 1) should be performed after rubbing Zusanli (ST 30). Held the big toe of the right foot with the fingers of the right hand to expose the sole of the foot. Then rub Yongquan (KI 1), a point in the front 1/3 of the sole, with Laogong (PC 8) or the centre of the palm of the left hand for 50 times. Do the same for the Yongquan (KI 1) point at the left foot. This can prevent flaring-up of fire and tonify the water.

(4) The diet should be controlled during qigong exercise, especially the fatty, greasy and spicy food or food made from flour. Sexual activities should also be controlled.

9. 1. 2 Qigong therapy in Chao's Syndrome of Diabetes

Chao Yuanfang, an eminent physician of the Sui Dynasty, recorded a therapy by dispersing and inducing method of qigong in his monograph *Treatise on Causes and Symptoms of Diseases*, which is applicable to the upper type of diabetes marked by polydipsia and dysuria. Its mechanism lies in relieving thirst through distributing the lung-fluid.

Section One: Lying silently with the lumber bending upward to promote flow of qi

Procedures: Loose cloth and untie the belt to lie flat on one's back. The waist is hunged up with the coccygeal vertebrae supporting the bed. The two hands are placed naturally on the two sides of the body. Close the eyes slightly and promp the upper palate with the tongue. Breath deeply, evenly and long for 5 times and expand the lower abdomen during the respiration.

Section Two: Stirring in the mouth and swallowing saliva

Procedure: Following above, stir with the tongue up and down for 9 times and right and left for 9 times between the lips and teeth. Then gurgle 18 times. After that, the saliva produced is swallowed down at several times and induced to dantian. Then lie camlly for

207

several minutes.

Section Three: End the exercise slowly

Procedure: Following the above, stand up and have a slow walk outside the door in the place where the air is fresh, the trees are flourishing and the environment is silent. The walk contains 12 steps to 1000 steps in a relaxed state.

Notes:

(1) The method must not be applied after meal or at an empty stomach.

(2) Take a proper diet which is composed of various nutrients. Spicy, fatty and greasy foods or decayed or unclean foods should be avoided. Have a meal slowly and avoid going to bed right after eating.

9. 1. 3 Case Study

Case 1.

Zhao is a 58-year old female who was treated in qigong Rehabilitation Hospital of Beidaihe. Since 1977, she began to have polydipsia, polyphagia, polyuria and general weakness and was diagnosed as having diabetes in a local hospital after an examination showing blood sugar at an empty stomach being 16. 67 mmol/L and urine sugar (++++). After that she had been treated systemically and was administered D860, Jiangtangling, Xiaokewan, glyburide, Yu Quang Wan and Liuwei Dihuang Wan, etc. , along with the diet control. One year later, the dosage of the drugs are increased as no satisfactory effects occurred, which is also ineffective. As a result, she began to receive insulin by injection, 40 u each day. Observations made during the five years of using insulin showed that once the insulin was stopped , the sugar in the blood and urine would soon elevate and she become extremely lassitude and almost unable to walk. As the treatment given in the local hospital was not effective, She was transferred to The Qigong Rehabilitation Hospital of Beidaihe to undergo qigong therapy after she had been stayed in the local hospital

208

for 18 months.

The admission examination indicated her blood sugar was 10. 83 mmol/L and the urine sugar was(+ +) while treated with insulin. Then she was ordered to exercise Yiming Gong(Exercise for Improving Eyesight)and still treated with insulin. The method of qigong exercise she took is one kind of respiration named respiration with flexion and extension of the arms. In a short time, she felt the flow of qi in her arms, could accumulate and disperse qi in her body freely and was able to be disattracted. She also felt improved herself and the qualitative urine sugar test showed her improvement. With more exercise, the internal qi could be well coordinated with respiration and she could become more disattracted, which indicated her further improvement. As a result, the dosage of insulin was gradually decreased, she became energetic and her spirit was high 20 days later. The blood sugar was normal and the urine sugar test showed a negative result. Then insulin was stopped and she was discharged after having been observed for 20 days. (From *Effective Qigong Therapy of Modern China*).

Case 2.

Zhang was a 73-year old male whose blood sugar at an empty stomach was 10 mmol/L and the urine sugar(+ +) tested in a hospital for the sake of his polypesia, polyuria and general weakness. He was treated with insulin in the hospital which relieved his symptoms temperorily. Then, he took D860 to maintain the condition but the disease developed further. In 1970, the symptoms were aggravated and the blood sugar at an empty stomach reached 11. 2mmol/L and the urine sugar was(+ + +). The disease was not controlled until the May, 1982. At this time, his blood sugar at an empty stomach was 12. 78mmol/L and the urine sugar(+ + + +). He felt generally exhausted and have unsteady gait, blurred vision. Then he began the qigong therapy, but drugs as Jiangtang Ling was still applied in the initial. Two weeks later, the symptoms were somewhat relieved, but they would become severe and the blood sugar increased once Jiang-tang Ling was administed. Two months later, his symptoms were basically relieved, his sight improved and his strength enhanced. The blood sugar at an empty stomach decreased to 7. 33 mmol/L and the urine sugar test($\pm$) . From then on, Jiangtang Ling was gradually stopped. (From *Treatment of* 29 *kinds of Chronic Diseases with Qigong*, Page 80.)

9. 2 Acupuncture therapy

9. 2. 1 Selection of points according to syndromes

1) Diabetes in the upper-jiao

Therapeutic principle: Clearing heat from the lung and moistening dryness.

Points: From mainly The Taiyin Meridians of both hand and foot and the back shu points: Feishu(UB 13), Hegu(LI 4), Yuji(LU 10), Lianquan(RN 23), Zhaohai(KI 6) and Sanyinjiao(SP 6).

Manipulations: Moderate reduction and reinforcement.

Explanation: Feishu(UB 13) and Hegu(LI 4) were used to clear away heat from the upper-jiao to moisten the lung; Yuji(LU 10),the Shu point of the Lung Meridian, to clear lung-heat; Lianquan(RN 23) to clear heat, benefit the throat, promote the production of body fluid to relieve thirst; and Zhaohai(KI 6) and Sanyinjiao(SP 6), to nourish the kidney, the root of the yin-fluid of the body, to tonify the lung.

2) Diabetes in the middle-jiao

Therapeutic principle: clearing away heat from the stomach, nourishing yin and promoting production of body fluid.

Points: from maily the Ren Meridian, the Foot-Yangming Meridian and the Foot-Taiyin Meridian: Zhongwan(RN 12), Tianshu(ST 25), Dadu(SP 2), Xiangu(ST 43), Sanyinjiao(SP 6)and Taixi(KI 3).

Manipulations: Reduction.

210

Explanation: Zhongwan (RN 12), the mu point of the Stomach Meridian and the convergent point of the fu organs, was used together with Tianshu (ST 25) to promote flow of qi in the intestine; Dadu combined with Sanyinjiao (SP 6) to purge the spleen-heat; Xiangu to purge the stomach-heat; and the combined use of Sanyinjiao (SP 6) and Taixi (KI 3) can nourish the kidney-yin to moisten dryness.

3) Diabetes in the lower-jiao

Therapeutic principle: nourishing the kidney-yin.

Points: Mainly from the shu points on the back and the points of Foot-Shaoyin and Foot-Taiyin: Shenshu (UB 23), Taixi (KI 3), Sanyinjiao (SP 6), Zhaohai (KI 6).

Manipulation: reinforcement.

Explanation: The diabetes in the lower-jiao is ascribed to deficiency of the kidney-yin and the subsequent flaring-up of fire. So, Shenshu (UB 23) was used to replenish the kidney-qi; Taixi (KI 3) and Zhaohai (KI 6) to nourish the kidney-yin and clear the residue heat in the lower-jiao; and Sanyinjiao (SP 6), the meeting spot of the three yin meridians of the feet, to benefit the three yin.

4) Diabetes due to interior heat caused by yin-deficiency

Main manifestations: Dire thirst with preference for drink, polyphagia, frequent urination which may be as turbid as fat in appearance, emaciation, or constipation, or soreness and weakness of the loins and knees, dizziness, tinnitus, red tongue with little coating, thready or slippery pulse.

Therapeutic principle: Nourishing yin to clear away heat.

Points: Geshu (UB 17), Pishu (UB 20), Yishu, Shenshu (UB 23), Zusanli (ST 30), Quchi (LI 11), Taixi (KI 3).

Manipulation: Moderate reduction and reinforcement. Retaining the needle for 15 to 30 minutes after feeling of qi is got.

Explanation: Geshu (UB 17), Pishu (UB 20) and Shenshu (UB 23), the points on the back (a yang part of the body), were used to induce Yin to Yang so that the yin is nourished and the yang-heat is cleared; Zusanli(ST 30), the convergent point of the Stomach Meridian of Foot-Yangming, to induce the genuine qi to go upward and thus the body fluid is produced; and Quchi(LI 11) and Taixi(KI 3) to purge heat and nourish Yin.

5) Diabetes due to deficiency of yang-qi

Main manifestations: Thirst with preference for drinks, poor appetite, profuse urine, or anorexia accompanied with frequent urination which appears as turbid fluid, lassitude, aversion to cold and cold limbs, or dark complexion and dry ears, pale tongue with whitish and dry coating, thready and feeble pulse.

Therapeutic principle: Warming up yang and invigorating qi.

Points: Qihai(RN 6), Zhongwan(RN 12), Zusanli(ST 30), Diji (SP 8), Chize(LU 5), Sanyinjiao(SP 6).

Manipulation: Reinforcement. Retaining the needles more than 30 minutes after the feeling of qi is got.

Explanation: Qihai(RN 6) and Zhongwan(RN 12), the points located at the abdomen(a yin part of the body), were used to induce yin to yang to strengthen yang and tonify deficiency so that yang is generated and yin-cold is expelled; Diji(SP 8), Sanyinjiao(SP 6) and Chize(LU 5), to help to promote the transformation and transportation of the spleen and stomach as well as the distribution of the lung-qi to invigorate and activate yang-qi.

6) Complications

Palpitation: Neiguan(PC 6), Shanzhong(RN 17), Xinshu(UB 15).

Constipation: Tianshu(ST 25), Dachangshu(UB 25), Zhigou(TJ 6), Zhaohai(KI 6).

Diarrhea: Tianshu(ST 25), Qihai(RN 6), Pishu(UB 20), Shangjuxu(ST 37).

Frequent, urgent and painful urination: Pangguangshu(UB28), Zhongshu(DU 7), Yinlingquan(SP 9), Xingjian(LI 2), Taixi(KI 3).

212

Puriritis: Qugu(RN 2), Xialiao(UB 34), Xuehai(SP 10), Ligou (LI 5), Zhongfu(LU 1), Xingjian(LI 7).

Numbness or pain of limbs: Zhongwan(RN 12), Qihai(RN 6), Zusanli(ST 30). Add Jianyu(LI 15), Quchi(LI 11) and Hegu(LI 4) in case of pain of the upper limbs, and add Fengshi(GB 31), Yinshi(ST 33), Yanglingquan(GB 34) and Jiexi(ST 41) in case of pain of the lower limbs.

Night blindness or cataract: Ganshu(UB 18), Shenshu(UB 23), Taixi(KI 3), Guangming(GB 37), Fengchi(GB 20), Jingming(UB 1), Chengqi(ST 1), Taiyang(Extra).

9. 2. 2 Other Acupuncture therapy

1) Otopuncture

This is a method by needling specific points of the ears, which has a wide indications. The names of the ear points are named after their related indications. For example, the Heart, Liver, Spleen, Kidney, Pancreas and Endocrine can be used to treat the disorders of their corresponding tissues and organs. When a diabetic patient exhibits pain of the limbs, insomnia, restlessness and hyperhidrosis, he or she can be treated through ear-acupuncture with high effects. This therapy is especially effeetive for those with pain. Throughout history, miscellaneous records were made in the medical literature on the names of ear-points, their locations, functions and indications. In recent years, some new ear-points have been reported at home and abroad, only that their contents are not completely identical. In June, 1987, The West Pacific Branch of WHO discussed the schedule for standarization of the ear-points in the Conference on the Standarization of Acupoints held in Korea. The locations of the ear-points are shown on Fig. 1.

The commonly-used ear-points for diabetes are: Pancreas, Endocrine, Sanjiao, Ermigen, Shenmen, Heart and Liver. They are to be stimulated mildly with filiform needles, or by intradermal embedding of needles, or by pressing with vaccaria seeds. Usually 3 — 5

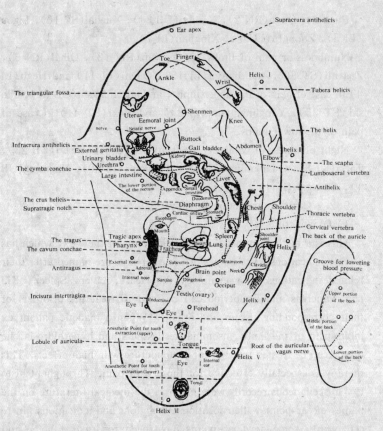

Fig. 1

points of one ear are used and the needles retained for 20 minutes, once every other day. One course of treatment consists of 10 treatments. The vaccaria seeds used to press points are retained on one ear for three days, after that they are applied to the other ear.

2) Acu-injection therapy

Apply the liquid of Hong Hua(Flos Carthami), Dang Gui(Radix Angelicae Sinensis), and Huang Qi(Radix Astragali seu Hedysari) or saline glucose or small dose of insulin to inject the following points: Feishu(UB 13), Pishu(UB 20), Weishu(UB 21), San-jiaoshu(UB 22), Shenshu(UB 23), Quchi(Li 11), Zusanli(ST 30), and Sanyinjiao(SP 6), 2 to 4 points each time, 0.5—2 ml for one point, once every two days. Five treatments form a course of treatment.

3) Electro-needle-therapy

Points: Yishu, Feishu(UB 13), Pishu(UB 20), Shenshu(UB 23), Zusanli(ST 30) and Sanyinjiao(SP 6). 2 to 4 of the points are selected each time. After feeling of qi is gained by needling, connect the needles with the Electro- Needling Instrument and stimuli the points for 15 minutes with intense wave. Once every other day.

4) Plum-blossom-needle therapy

Knock 7 to 10 areas beside the spinal column, once every day or every other day. One course of treatment lasts 5 to 10 treatments.

5) Warming moxibustion

Points: ① Qihai(RN 6), Guanyuan(RN 4), Lieque(LU 7), Zhaohai(KI 6), Shuidao(ST 28); ② Mingmen(DU 4), Shenshu (UB 23), Huiyin(RN 1), Zhongji(RN 3), Weiyang(UB 39). The points of the two groups are to be selected alternately and one moxing treatment lasts 15 to 20 minutes, once every other day, and 10 treatments form one course of treatment.

6) Moxibustion with ginger

Points to be selected include 8 groups: ① Zusanli(ST 30), Zhong-wan(RN 12); ② Mingmen(DU 4), Shenzhu(DU 12), Pishu(UB 20); ③ Qihai(RN 6), Mingmen(DU 4); ④ Jizhong(DU 6), Shen-shu(UB 23) ⑤ Huagai(RN 20), Liangmen(ST 21); ⑥ Dazhui (DU 14), Ganshu(UB 18); ⑦Xingjian(LI 7), Zhongji(RN 3), Fuai(SP 16); ⑧ Geshu(UB 17), Feishu(UB 13), Shenshu(UB 23). One group of the above is used each time, and the ginger slice is 3 to 4 mm thick and 1.5cm in diameter. The moxa cone is 1.5 cm in diameter and 2cm high, weighing 0.5g. 10 to 30 times are required for each point and once every other day, 50 days forms one course of treatment.

7) Warming moxibustion with orange peel

Points selected include: Yemen(SJ 2), Yangchi(TJ 5), Yishu, and Sanjiaoshu(UB 22). Cut a fresh or a soaked dry orange peel into the slice 2 cm in size with a 1 cm long cut edge. When the needle is inserted, manipulate it with moderate reduction and reinforcement. Then insert the segment of moxa cone into the hole of the needle,cover the slice of the orange peel over the body of the needle and close the slice to the skin. Then put a hard paper between the slice and the skin. Ignite the end near the skin of the moxa cone. Once every day and 10 treatments form one course of treatment.

Notes:

(1) Acupuncture is effective for the mild and moderate types of diabetes. Drug therapy should be combined in case of chronic or critical patients.

(2) Diabetes is a chronic disease, thus the course of acupuncture therapy is long. Usually 3 to 4 months is necessary to acquire the marked therapeutic effect, and early stoppage of acupuncture should be avoided.

(3) Patients of diabetes usually have lowered resistance and are susceptible to secondary infection. So before needling, strict disinfection is required in order to prevent infection.

9. 2. 3 Case Study

Xu is a 50 years old male who was admitted on April 14, 1984 with a history of polydipeia, polyuria and obvious emaciation for two weeks. Two weeks before, he was found to have thirst, polydipsia and polyuria, lassitude at times, insomnia with dream- disturbed sleep, and obvious emaciation. His appetite was still good. He went to seek medical care in a hospital where tests showed that his blood sugar was 13. 4mmol/L and the urine sugar(++++). He was treated with Youjiangtang and Xiaoke Wan, which relieved the symptoms but the urine sugar still remained the same. So he was admitted

216

to the hospital.

On physical examination, he has a clear mind, sallow complexion, emaciation, and scattered red neves. The nerve system showed no abnormality and his heart and lung were normal. The spleen and liver were also normal in size. His tongue was red with thin and yellow fur, and his pulse is deep and thready. The blood sugar at an empty stomach was 11. 1mmol/ l, and the urine sugar was (++++).

Impression: Diabetes.

Therapeutic principle: Nourishing yin to clear away heat, moistening dryness and promoting the production of body fluid.

Selection of points: Lieque (LU 7), Zhaohai (KI 6), Zhongwan (RN 12), Sanyinjiao (SP 6), Shenshu (UB 23), Geshu (UB 17) and Feishu (UB 13).

Manipulations: Needled Lieque (LU 7) 1 cun deep toward the elbows, and Zhaohai (KI 6) 0. 5 cun deep vertically, with reinforcement by rotating the points 1 minutes; Zhongwan (RN 12) 2 cun deep vertically with 1 minute of reduction by respiration and a feeling spreading over the whole abdomen; Sanyinjiao (SP 6) 1 cun deep vertically with 1 minute of reinforcement by rotating the needle; Shenshu (UB 23) 1. 5 cun deep vertically, Geshu (UB 17), Pishu (UB 20) and Feishu (UB 13) 1. 5 cun obliquely toward the vertebrate with 1 minute of reinforcement by rotating the needles and a feeling spread to the front. The above points were used twice a day and alternately in the morning and evening.

Three days later, the thirst was alleviated and the lassitude disappeared. The urine sugar was tested (+++) . 2 weeks later, the blood sugar at an empty stomach reduced to 8. 9 mmol/1 and the urine sugar (+), which were further reduced to 6. 4mmol/1 and ± respectively after 4 week's treatment. So, he was clinically cured and discharged. He was advised to control diet by himself.

Follow-up during the half a year after his discharge showed that his blood sugar was kept less than 8.3mmol/1 and urine sugar (++). (From *A Collection of Shi Xuemin's Clinical Experience of Acupuncture*)

9.3 Massage Therapy

9.3.1 Therapeutic manipulations

The patient is asked to take a proper position to expose the areas to be treated, the apply massage therapy to the head, abdomen, back and limbs respectively. Then precedures and the manipulations are as follows:

(1) Head: The chief selected manipulations include pressing, digital pressing, pushing, tapping, and vibrating. The main points selected are Chengjiang(RN 24), Duiduan(DU 27) and Pancreas(an ear point),and the compatible points are Fengchi(GB 20), Zanzhu(UB 2), Jingming(UB 1), Taiyang(Extra), Baihui(DU 20) and Shenmen(HT 7) and Endocrine of the ear(Fig. 2—Fig. 8).

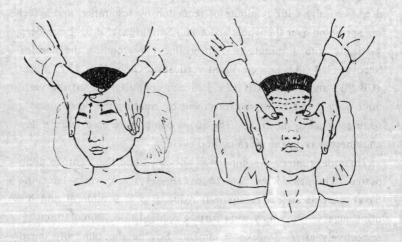

Fig. 2

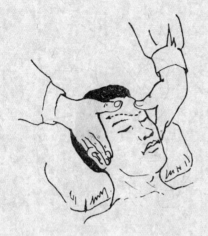

Fig. 3

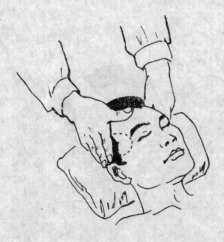

Fig. 4

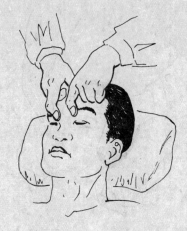

Fig. 5

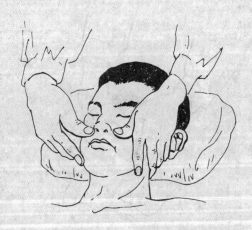

Fig. 6

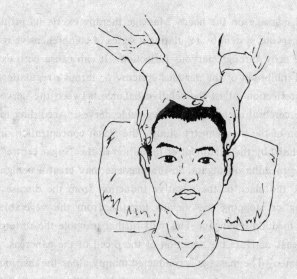

Fig. 7

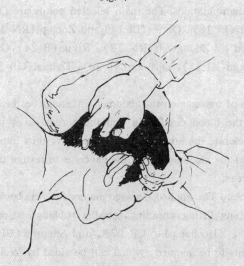

Fig. 8

221

Effects of massage on the head: Massage therapy exerts its influence on the nervous system by regulating a series of comprehensive reaction of the body through nervous reflection. It can cause both excitement and inhibition of the nervous system, or through regulating the nervous reflection adjust the relative balance between the nerve centre of the cerebral cortex and the vegetable nerves. According to the conclusion of the biochemistry study, the plasm concentration of sugar is regulated by the excitment or inhibition of the "sugar centre" located at the medulla oblangata. So the massage may creat a benign focus to take the place of the negative induction from the disease, thus reducing or stopping the vicious impulse from the vegetable nerve to the medulla oblangata. This will further promote the restore of the pancreas, activate the secretion of the β cell of the pancreas.

(2) Abdomen: The massage is conducted mainly along the distribution of the colon with pushing, grasping, palm-rubbing or digital pressing manipulations. The main selected points are Qihai(RN 6), Zhangmen(LI 13), Qimen(LI 14) and Zhongji(RN 3), which can be assisted by Zhongwan(RN 12), Riyue(B 24), Guanyuan(RN 4), Henggu(KI 11), Qichong(ST 30), Daimai(GB 26), etc(Fig. 9).

Effects of massage on the abdomen: Massage on the abdomen may promote the blood circulation and the peristalsis of the gastrointestine, accelerate the absorption and digestion, thus improving the nutrients and the blood supply to the pancreas to restore the function of the pancreas.

(3) Back: The applied massage methods on the back include pushing, grasping, lifting, kneading, pressing, rubbing and padding. Feishu (UB 13), Xiaochangshu(UB 27), and Shenshu(UB 23) are the main pionts to be adopted, which can be aided by Weishu(UB 21), Sanjiaoshu(UB 22)(Fig. 10).

Effect of massage on the back: As there are many points located at the two sides of the spinal column, massage on the meridians beside

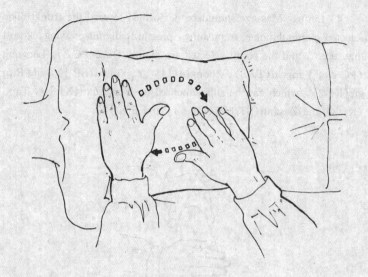

Fig. 9

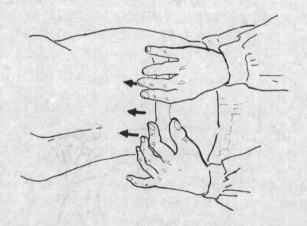

Fig. 10

the spinal column, especially the chiropractic, can strengthen the reflection of the spinal nerve. When some special points are selected,
the quick restore of the pancreas can be expected.

223

(4) Limbs: Massage should be performed toward the trunk. The selected manipulations are pushing, pressing, digital pressing, kneading, etc. , and the points selected are mainly Quze(PC 3), Laogong (PC 8), Yangchi(TJ 5), Zhongfu(LU 1), Yinbai(SP 1), and Rangu(KI 2), which can be supplemented by Yongquan(KI 1), Taixi (KI 3) and Zusanli(ST 30)(Fig. 11 and Fig. 12).

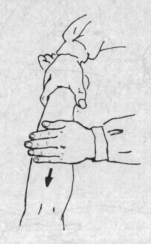

Fig. 11

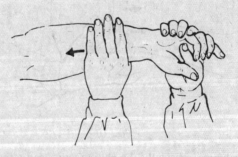

Fig. 12

Effect of massage on the limbs: Massage on the limbs can increase the back flow of blood to the heart, improve blood circulation, especially the microcirculation of the limbs. So it can promote the tissue metabolism and accelerate the absorption and application of sugar in the cells, which helps to regulate the osmotic pressure inside and outside the cells and improve the renel function indirectly to accelerate the discharge of the waste in the tissues. Meanwhile, it can also prevent or reduce over decomposition of protein and fat so that the production of the ketone bodies and break the viscious cycle of metabolism, laying a firm basis for the restore of the function of the pancreas.

Clinical observation indicates that general massage has the effect of lowering down blood sugar and urine sugar and alleviating symtoms.

(5) Course of treatment: Once or twice a day, each treatment lasting 15 to 20 minutes. One course of treatment consists of 10 to 30 days' treatments.

9. 3. 2. Selection of Masso-points in accordance with syndromes

Diabetes is divided into three types: that in the upper-jiao, middle-jiao and lower-jiao. The diabetes in the upper-jiao is ascribed to the lung-heat, that in the middle-jiao to stomach-heat, and that in the lower-jiao, to the kidney-deficiency. Patients of different types may have different manifestations, polydipsia, polyphagia or polyuria, which may not occur simultaneously.

(1) Diabetes in the upper-jiao:

Therapeutic method: Clearing heat and moistening the lung, promoting the production of body fluid to relieve thirst.

Points of selection: Shaoshang (LU 11), Hegu (LI 4), Daimai (GB 26), Chengjiang (RN 24), Rangu (Ki 2), Yinbai (SP 1), Feishu (UB 13), Xinshu (UB 15), Weishu (UB 21), Dibazhuixia (Extra), Laogong (PC 8), Gongsun (SP 4), etc.

(2) Diabetes in the middle-jiao:

Therapeutic method: Purging the stomach-heat to reserve yin-fluid.

Points of selection: Baihui(DU 20), Zhongwan(RN 12), Riyue (BL 24), Guanyuan(RN 4), Xinshu(UB 15), Weishu(UB 21), Pishu(UB 20), Zusanli(ST 30), Sanyinjiao(SP 6), Yangchi(TJ 5), etc.

(3) Diabetes in the lower-jiao:

Therapeutic method: Nourishing the kidney-yin and promoting the production of body fluid to clear away heat.

Points of selection: Zhangmen(LI 13), Xiaochangshu(UB 27), Shenshu(UB 23), Zhongji(RN 3), Shuidao(ST 28), Duiduan(DU 27), Sanjiaoshu(UB 22), Zhongfu(LU 1), Sanyinjiao(SP 6), Endocrine(ear-point), Shenmen(HT 7), Henggu(KI 11), etc.

(4) Points for complications

① Headache: Select Yintang(Extra), Qianding(DU 21), Touwei (ST 8) and Shangxing(DU 23) for pain of the forehead, Baihui(DU 20), Qianding(DU 21) and Houding(DU 19) for pain at the top, Fengchi(GB 20), Tianzhu(UB 10) and Xinshu(UB 15) for pain of the occipital region, and Taiyang(Extra) and Touwei(ST 8) for pain of the sides of the head.

② Lassitude: Select Zusanli(ST 30), Quchi(LI 11), Hegu(LI 4), Xingjian(LI 7), Gaohuang, and Dazhui(DU 14).

③ Diarrhea: Select Zusanli(ST 30), Tianshu(ST 25), Neiguan (PC 6), Qihai(RN 6), Sanyinjiao(SP 6), Shenque(RN 8), Weizhong(UB 40) and quick strong stimuli.

④ Constipation: Zusanli(ST 30), Tianshu(ST 25), Yanglingquan(GB 34) and Taibai(SP 3).

⑤ Pain of the upper limbs: Select Neiguan(PC 6), Waiguan(TJ 5), Quchi(LI 11), and Hegu(LI 4) for pain of the forearm, and Quchi(LI 11), Jianjing(GB 21) and Jianyu(LI 15) for pain of the upper arms. For paralysis of the upper limbs, the above-mentioned points should be used alternately with strong stimuli.

⑥ Pain of the lower limbs with dyskenisia: Select Yangfu(GB

226

38), Sanyinjiao(SP 6), Yinlingquan(SP 9),Yanglingquan(GB 34) and Zusanli(ST 30) for pain of the lower legs, Biguan(ST 31), Huantiao(GB 30) and Yanglingquan(GB 34) for pain of the thign, and Kunlun(UB 60), Zhaohai(KI 6) and Rangu(KI 2) for pain of the soles. For paralysis of the lower limbs, the above points should be used alternately with quick strong stimuli.

⑦ Edema of the lower limbs: Select Shangjuxu(ST 37), Xiajuxu (ST 39), Sanyinjiao(SP 6) and Zusanli(ST 30).

⑧ Frequent urination: Select Qihai(RN 6), Zhongji(RN 3), Guanyuan (RN 4), Sanyinjiao (SP 6), Duiduan (DU 27) and Shuidao(ST 28).

9. 3. 3 Self-massage therapy

(1) Kneading the back shu points: Hold a fist to knead the muscles on the bilateral sides of the spinal column from the prominence downwards. Yishu, the point beside the 8th vertebral process, should be specially kneaded. This is repeated several times, which lasts about three minutes. If a hot sensation is produced, the therapeutic effect would be even satisfactory.

(2) Kneading and pressing the back: With the dorsum of one hand, knead and press one side of the back until a hot feeling is felt. Then, with the dorsum of the other hand, knead and press the other side of the back. This is done alternatively for two minutes.

(3) Rubbing the abdomen: Rub gently the abdomen counterclockwise. At the polnts Guanyuan (RN- 4) and Qihai (RN- 6), exert more strength. This is repeated $100-200$ times.

(4) Digiting and kneading the points Neiguan(PC 6), Zusanli(ST 30) and Shousanli: This manipulation should be down on the three points respectively for one minute.

(5) Kneading and pressing Yongquan(KI 1) point: Rubbing the two hands to produce heat, then knead and press Yongquan.

(6) Tap the lumbus and back gently with moderate strength with the two fists. When soreness, distension and hotness are felt by the

patient, end the manipulation.

9. 3. 4 Case study

Guo is a 48-year old male who was admitted to be treated with massage for his diabetes. Case number: 72162.

The clinical manifestations include thirst with excessive drinking, polyphagia, dizziness, lassitude, obvious weight loss. He had been treated with diet therapy and common insulin, 60 u per day, and his urine glucose was 48 grams in 24 hours. After the first massage treatment, the dose of insulin was reduced to 40 u per day which was further reduced to 8 u per day after one week of treatment. Two weeks later the insulin was stopped after fourteen treatments, the patient had a good appetite and experienced the relief of his symptoms, and his weight was increased by 1. 5 kilogram. The symptoms disappeared after thirty treatments, the blood sugar decreased to 8. 06mmol/L, and the urine glucose was negative. Reexamination half a year later showed that his blood sugar was 6. 22mmol/L, the urine glucose was kept negative, and his weight was increased from 53 kg to 65 kg. Follow-up in the following three years indicated that the disease was stablised and no recurrence was experienced.

糖尿病中医治疗

陈金锭　编著

翻译　孙英葵　周树辉

英文审校　路玉宾

*

山东科学技术出版社出版

（中国济南玉函路 16 号　邮政编码 250002）

外文印刷厂印刷

中国国际图书贸易总公司发行

（中国北京车公庄西路 35 号）

（北京邮政信箱第 399 号　邮政编码 100044）

1994 年（大 32）　1 版 1 次

5331—1459

定价：30.00元

14E2794P

Editor in Charge   Li Chuanhou
First Edition 1994
ISBN 7-5331-1459-0

Treatment of Diabetes
with Traditional Chinese Medicine
Written By Chen Jinding
Translated By Sun Yingkui
Zhou Shuhui
English Revised By Lu Yubin
Published By **Shandong Science and Technology Press**
16 Yuan Road, Jinan, CHINA   250002
Printed By Shandong Xin Hua Printing House
Distributed By China International Book Trading Corporation
35 Chegongzhuang Xilu, Beijing   100044, China
P. O. Box 399, Beijing, China
Printed in the People's Republic of China